Praise for 5(

"Ron Whitchurch has the observational wit and insight of a modern day Mark Twain and the eyebrows and mustache to match."

— **Koco Eaton**, MD, ABOS, Team Physician, Tampa Bay Rays

"This is an extraordinary book which brilliantly and compellingly conveys to the lay person the day-to-day workings of the operating room. What is amazing is how one person could have seen and experienced so much. The chapters are interesting, insightful, hilarious, sometimes sardonic yet compassionate, demonstrating the stress, sorrow, pathos and joy of dealing with patients and families under the best and worst of situations."

— **Kevin M. Sweeney**, MD, board-certified neurosurgeon, former chief of Neurosurgery of Mease hospitals in Dunedin and Clearwater, Florida

"Lessons learned — lives saved is a consistent theme in Ron's nitty-gritty personal recollection of his vast professional experiences as a CRNA. You'll get an incredible narrative of true life tales straight from the horse's mouth and some of those will knock your socks off!!"

— **Carol Hathaway**, BSN, RN, CNOR

"I loved reading this wonderful collection of triumphs, tragedies, near misses, and so many funny situations in the OR. Ron is an anesthesia historian, a keen observer of the quirks and ironies of life in surgery and a colorful storyteller. A fascinating and clearly explained glimpse at the world on the other side of the drapes."

— **Antonio J. Gayoso**, MD, ASPS, ASAPS

"This collection embodies skill, technology, compassion, personal relations, drama and humor. Ron's recall and vivid recording of his most memorable experiences were a delight to read. His innumerable patients have had the benefit of a truly knowledgeable, skillful and caring practitioner."

— **David B. Fitch**, CRNA (retired)

"Ever wonder what happens in the OR after the anesthetist says 'Have a nice nap. See you when you wake up?' Ron Whitchurch's true stories will take you into the operating room in a way that makes you feel you are there. A clear picture of his compassion, his caring for others, and his wonderful sense of humor shine through. I highly recommend his book."

— **Claudette Holly**, RN, Or Supervisor, Director of Perioperative Services

"This memoir is fun and fact-filled — typical of the author, riveting and mind boggling and kept me spellbound. A very enjoyable trip down memory lane through the retrospectroscope. This book is one of a kind, just like its author."

— **John Danner**, CRNA (retired)

"This book will not put you to sleep! Ron's vivid accounts introduce the reader into the operating room and into the horrifying, the heartbreaking, and the humorous cases performed."

— **Ray Shefland**, CRNA, RC, Shefland Anesthesia Ltd., 46-year career of providing rural anesthesia and mentee of Ron Whitchurch

"These are amazing, authentic memories of as broad a scope of cases as one could imagine, stories that could not have been made up and told with insight, transparency and an indomitable sense of humor. Such a rich experience is a must read for anyone who has had or is interested in anesthesia."

— **Sondra Shields**, MD, Mayo Clinic trained, Board Certified in Anesthesiology and Pain Management

"This memoir shares a multitude of experiences Ron has witnessed, from the many miracles to the highs and lows of the anesthesia world. I worked with Ron before he retired. One of the many God-given talents that always amazed me was how he could calm a pre-operative patient of their anxieties. *50 Years in the OR* shows both the serious and humorous side of medicine."

— **Donna Tessier**, RN, BSN, CRNI, CAPA

"This is a fun, informative and revealing book that will be enjoyed by medical professionals as well as non-medical readers."

— **Dwight Valentine**, MD, President and Managing Partner of Gulfcoast Anesthesia Partners, Vice President and Board Member of Greater Florida Anesthesiologists, a division of Sheridan/Envision Anesthesia

"As a busy OB/GYN, I worked directly with Ron on many cases in the OR and OB unit. Along with being an excellent and compassionate CRNA, I've known Ron to have a very well developed sense of humor and ability to tell a good story. In this book, Ron takes the reader behind the scenes to share his personal episodes of drama, humor and stress in his anesthesia career managing the routine and completely unexpected. From hunting accidents to childbirth, Minnesota to Florida — life and death unfold."

— **Thomas G. Walter**, MD, FACOG, Diplomate, American Board of Obstetrics and Gynecology, Fellow, American College of Obstetricians and Gynecologists

"I have been on the other side of medicine for Ron. I have been part of Ron's team — as his cancer specialist — as he continues to battle Multiple Myeloma. Our journey has shown me a great deal about Ron and it has been and continues to be a joyful experience. Ron will keep you on your toes, educate you and make you laugh. I hope that the story of his life's work does the same for you."

— **Kenneth Shain**, MD, PhD, Department of Malignant Hematology Oncology, Moffitt Cancer Center

"Take a trip into the OR and sit with Ron as though it is happening and he will share his stories. You will feel what it is like to experience the tremendous responsibility that the anesthetist has. You also will gain much respect for the men and women that carry that responsibility with every patient. Enjoy this remarkable journey that Ron has had, as he most certainly has."

— **Peter Nelson**, Mora, Minnesota

"I am in awe of this book and of the years that Ron worked. This is a great read from My First Case until Room 4737. CRNAs will enjoy reading this, and nurses interested in anesthesia will find a book that most assuredly will make them want to be a part of this profession. Read this book — you will enjoy it immensely."

— **Sandra Kilde**, CRNA (retired), EdD, MA, BA, past Director of the Minneapolis School of Anesthesia

"When Ron came to our group we received a loyal friend, a colleague and a patient advocate, not to mention his intellectual levity that provided a measure of escape from the daily stress of the job. Ron and I provided thousands of anesthetics over the course of many years (some easy and some quite complex), but our patients' safety was always our primary goal. I always knew that I could count on Ron to represent our group in a professional manner amongst his peers, patients and hospital staff. I am so grateful to have met him and shared all the fun and maybe scary times together."

— **Jan Duvoisin**, MD, Board Certified Anesthesiologist, Morton Plant Mease Hospitals, Surgery Partners at Westchase, Medical Village of TGH and Sarasota

50 Years in the OR

True Stories of Life, Loss, and Laughter
While Giving Anesthesia

Ron Whitchurch

Published by Loon Lake Press
www.loonlakepress.com

Editor: David Aretha
Cover and Interior Design: Deana Riddle, BookStarter

ISBN 978-1-7360650-0-6 (paperback)
ISBN 978-1-7360650-1-3 (e-book)

Printed in the United States of America

"Giving anesthesia is basically many long hours of boredom punctuated by moments of sheer terror!"

— Bill Ritter

Dedicated to the memory of my dear, sainted mother

Katherine Jean Smith Whitchurch

And to the three Chiefs of Anesthesia I worked for during my career:

Bill Ritter, Jean Follman, and *Dwight Valentine*

Contents

Acknowledgements   1

Foreword   3

Preface   5

1. My First Case   9

2. The ACDF   11

3. The Empty O2 Tank   17

4. The Ladies' Man   21

5. The White Mustang   23

6. The Back Booth   25

7. Poor Bob   27

8. The Bet   29

9. Two Interesting Patients   31

10. Two Neurosurgery Stories   33

11. Three Tattoo Stories   35

12. The Diamond Ring   39

13. An Atheist   41

14. The Arm Block   43

15. The Hiccups   47

16. The Elevator   49

17. Brushing Teeth   51

18. Train Tracks   55

19. "I Resent That"   59

20. The Chick Table   61

21. Esophageal Varicies   63

22. Farm Accident   65

23. The Mixer   67

24. Popeye   69

25. Coffee in the Locker Room   71

26. Knock Me Out   73

27. Two Carotid Stories   75

28. Worried I won't Wake UP   79

29. The Thermostat   81

30. The Wrong Room   83

31. The Snowplow   85

32. Janie   89

33. The Horse Bite   93

34. Anesthesia Allergy   95

35. Baseball Player   97

36. Dead Battery   99

37. The Queen   103

38. Helping With the AAA   107

39. Motorcycle Head Injury   109

40. The Supraglottic Tumor   111

41. The Specimen Jar   115

42. Innovar Hypo   117

43. Two Tourniquet Stories   121

44. The Prep   125

45. New Anesthesia Machine   127

46. Crazy Days   129

47. The Housekeeper   131

48. Incarcerated Hernia   133

49. The Reflex   135

50. Two Car Crash Stories   137

51. The Dentures   141

52. Holiday Prescription Refill   143

53. Resuscitation   145

54. Unusual Delivery   147

55. Two Blood Transfusion Stories   149

56. The Shoulder Block   153

57. Bran Muffin   155

58. Bottled Water   157

59. Craniotomy Insufflation   159

60. The Gas Sampling Line   163

61. Tonsillectomy Experience   165

62. Frozen Buttocks   167

63. Sunflower Seeds 169

64. Pierre-Robin 171

65. Queasy Husband 173

66. Tonsillectomy Tooth 175

67. "Let Her Die" 177

68. Bad Taste 179

69. The Gold Grill 181

70. Rock Star 183

71. Linen Cart 185

72. Grouse Hunter 187

73. Unusual C-Section 191

74. The Bezoar 193

75. Perforated Bowel 195

76. Squirt in the Face 197

77. The ACL Repair 201

78. Omphalocele 205

79. Too Fat 207

80. Skin Wheal 209

81. The Observer 211

82. The Rebreathing Bag 213

83. Lawsuit and Expert Witness 217

84. MH 225

85. Mildred 229

86. Nursery   231

87. Multiple Personalities   233

88. Faux Pas   235

89. Speech Impediment   237

90. Graduate Student   239

91. Rigid Bronchoscopy   241

92. Ugly Doctor   245

93. An Alcoholic's Cure   247

94. Donor   249

95. Three Veterinary Stories   253

96. Over and Back   259

97. Heimlich Maneuver   263

98. My Old Chief CRNA   265

99. HIV Epidural   269

100. Bleeding Tonsil   271

101. Deer Hunting Gunshot Injuries   275

102. Engine Block   277

103. The '63 Ford Pickup   279

104. Foreign Bodies   281

105. Car Wreck   283

106. Demerol Anesthesia   285

107. Old Soldier Hip Fracture   289

108. The Art Gallery   291

109. Alcohol Infusion   293

110. Three Stories Before My Shift at the Hospital   295

111. Angel's Visit   301

112. Room #4737   305

Glossary   309

Acknowledgements

I would like to acknowledge and sincerely thank all of the remarkable people who helped me make this long-time-in-coming memoir possible.

My dear wife Lonnette, a former high school English teacher and speech coach, who was by my side offering invaluable guidance as I wrote this book. She did the initial edit of each story, making them interesting and readable, and gave me continual enthusiastic encouragement.

David Aretha, who edited my manuscript three times, gave me excellent advice on syntax and grammar and was always available for the multitude of questions I had.

My publishing team:

Deana Riddle, who designed the beautiful book cover and interior and helped publish this book in all the formats readers like to use.

Jeremy Avenarius, who constructed my gorgeous websites, designed the pretty loon logo and made Loon Lake Press available to the world.

Martha Bullen, without whom this book could never have gotten off the ground. With her vast knowledge and experience Martha worked tirelessly editing, suggesting chapter placements, putting me in touch with the experts I'd need for each aspect of publishing, directing me to the web tools needed to market my book and being the general manager for the entire complex project.

And a special thanks to all my friends, relatives, coworkers, supervisors and the physicians I worked with over the years for their support and encouragement, without which I may never have had the impetus to even start or complete this manuscript.

Foreword

I first met Ron Whitchurch when he came to work with our group of anesthesia providers. Ron had already had many years of anesthesia experience behind him, and many more to come with our group. Our group was the last group Ron was a part of and he was with us for sixteen years until his retirement.

As Ron has almost fifty years of experience in anesthesia, he has many stories and anecdotes about the growth of our profession and instances to which he has been privy. He will take you from his basic training (when we mostly used a manual blood pressure cuff, a stethoscope and a finger on the pulse) to today where we do complex cases with better monitoring than was used on the first space launch.

He wrote this book to share his experiences as his career evolved from a small town in Bemidji, Minnesota to an urban group of thirty-five providers in Florida so that readers could appreciate how complex a nurse anesthetist's job is and to share some of the highlights and most memorable moments.

As I also trained four decades ago, I can relate to how things have changed as anesthesia has become safer. Of course, this has come about because as the saying goes, "Good judgment comes from bad experience and bad experience comes from bad judgment." As you read this book, remember that anesthesia is not only a science but an art to make it look effortless.

Ron always had stories to share at the table in the break room. And he frequently would make friends with people passing by and soon would know their whole history. He writes as he speaks, and so the stories are short, often humorous, but always in truth. I think you will enjoy these stories and while they may not alleviate any of the stress of any future surgery, at least you will know the strides we have made to keep you safe and waking up happy.

Jean Follman
Chief CRNA, St. Petersburg, FL

Preface

Nurse anesthetists have been administering anesthesia for over a hundred years starting in the nineteenth century. They usually picked up their techniques from a surgeon or one of his assistants and then taught a few of the other nurses how to do it. But in 1889 Alice Magaw, considered the Mother of Nurse Anesthesia, established a formal anesthesia department at the Mayo Clinic in Rochester, Minnesota where visitors could go sit in a gallery to watch their expert administration of anesthesia. Alice's department, the Mayo Clinic program for Nurse Anesthesia, became the foremost in the world. In 1936 Dr. George W. Crile, one of America's famous surgeons, said of nurse anesthetists, "I think this movement is one of the most beneficent movements we have seen in the whole field of operative surgery." (Dr Crile was quoted in Watchful Care: A History of America's Nurse Anesthetists by Marianne Bankert.)

Modern-day nurses go through some fairly rigorous schooling and training to become a Certified Registered Nurse Anesthetist (CRNA). They need a Bachelor of Science degree in nursing (BSN), need to have passed their respective state nursing boards and need to have two years of critical care nursing experience before they can be considered for admittance to any of the nurse anesthesia programs. The current programs consist of three years of classroom and supervised clinical practice, and upon graduation they receive a master's degree and are qualified to sit for the national board exam to become a CRNA. In the near future the programs will bestow graduate anesthetists with a DNP (Doctor of Nursing Practice).

Statistics show that more than one-half of all the anesthetics administered in the United States are given by CRNAs. Many times they work in rural areas where they may be the only provider, or they might work in a larger hospital setting with a mixed practice of CRNAs and anesthesiologists. CRNAs are really the unsung heroes of the hospital world. Their backgrounds enable them to be familiar with almost every patient care or related department in the hospital and almost all the techniques and therapeutics that go with them. They can make beds or successfully administer anesthesia for a complicated brain surgery and everything in between.

I was drawn to nurse anesthesia from observing them in action as an orderly in the recovery room back in the 1960s at Northwestern Hospital in

Minneapolis. I was a student at the University of Minnesota at the time majoring in mathematics, but after three years I gave it up and completely changed directions. I went into a three-year, hospital-based registered nursing program, and after graduation enrolled in the Minneapolis School of Anesthesia. At that time anesthesia school was only eighteen months, and at graduation we all received a diploma and took our national boards to become a CRNA.

In 1971 I went to work in Bemidji, which is a small town in northern Minnesota, with one other CRNA. It was a one hundred-bed hospital that served a large surrounding area including two large Native American reservations. The two of us did all the anesthesia for scheduled surgery and emergency call, which we split 50/50. One week I was on call Monday, Tuesday, Friday, Saturday, Sunday, and the next week my call was Wednesday and Thursday. There were four general surgeons, two ophthalmologists, one urologist, one obstetrician/gynecologist and a few general practice doctors who did surgery regularly. Our daily surgeries ran anywhere from three to ten cases per day in three operating rooms.

The scheduled cases were pretty average ones: hernia repairs, gall bladders, gynecologic, etc., on mostly healthy patients but occasionally we would do a big vascular case like an elective abdominal aneurysm repair. The call cases were something else entirely. Most days on call it was work all day doing scheduled cases and all night doing emergency ones. We got almost every kind of emergency and trauma imaginable, from shootings, stabbings, beatings, and car wrecks to appendicitis, ectopic pregnancies, bowel obstructions, fish hooks in various body parts, and fractures. And, during deer hunting season in November, all the big city hunters would converge on our north woods and fill the emergency room regularly with some of the most bizarre injuries imaginable.

Administering anesthesia to patients for procedures was much different in the 1970s. In those days, we only worried about bringing bacteria into the OR ourselves and transmitting it to the patients. We weren't worried about the patients bringing a deadly disease to us. If the patient was sick with a cold or the flu, they just put off surgery until they were recovered. And, if a patient came in with an infected wound, it was debrided and they were treated with antibiotics. If they were in isolation because of a staph infection, we just put on a gown, gloves and mask when we brought them to surgery and after the case took them straight back to their isolation room and the OR they'd been in was wiped down with disinfectant.

Then in the early '80s the AIDS epidemic presented itself. Everybody in healthcare was frightened by it because we saw patients in various stages of the disease, some of whom were near death, and there was no apparent treatment or cure for it. Extreme caution was taken when starting patients' IVs, giving injections, and being around any of their bodily fluids. All patients were queried about whether they had AIDS or HIV but not everyone knew if they might have it, so we had to assume they did until proven otherwise. Also, in the early days of the disease, banked blood wasn't able to be tested for it and some unfortunates got the disease from a transfusion. Finally, HIV testing was perfected, effective antiretroviral drugs became available and healthcare workers calmed down quite a bit, but the precautions they had acquired stayed in place.

Now forward to 2020 and the COVID-19 virus pandemic. Healthcare workers are all but panicked by it because not only can it be spread by bodily fluids, it is also airborne. And it's all over the news showing some of the worst case scenarios with even healthy young people getting it and not surviving. Extreme precautions need to be taken by healthcare workers and caregivers so as not to become infected themselves. Anesthesia providers are particularly at risk because of their proximity to the surgical patient's airway, and some anesthesia departments have developed special teams wearing HAZMAT suits to perform all intubations and extubations.

Surgical schedules have been drastically altered too. At first hospitals closed down elective procedures completely, and then they allowed only emergency surgery and same day surgery with an hour between cases for room cleaning. As ICUs filled up, some anesthesia personnel were pulled from the department to help them out. Numerous staff members got COVID-19 infections which limited a department's resources and made for very long, stressful shifts for the remaining personnel. The COVID-19 virus has altered almost every aspect of healthcare and it doesn't look as if it will change anytime soon. The world's only hope in combating this disease is for an effective vaccine to be developed along with the availability of widespread rapid result testing. I think many of the new techniques and procedures that have been developed in the process will also remain in place forever.

I stayed in that little northern Minnesota town until 1987 when the bitter cold winters (occasionally 30 below zero) and overwhelming emergency call started to wear me out. I moved to the Tampa Bay area of Florida and worked with a large mixed group of anesthesiologists and CRNAs until I retired in November 2018. Looking back, I can honestly say that I loved every minute of my career and would do it all over again if I could.

The stories and events in this book are all true, but I have altered the names and dates in some cases for obvious reasons.

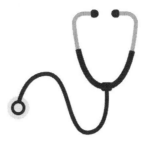

1. My First Case

"Ronald, I want you to go into room four and help Doctor Johnson, because he is doing a very interesting case right now and could use some help," said Dr. Irving Greenfield, chief of anesthesia at the Hennepin County hospital in downtown Minneapolis. It was my first morning of clinical practice with the Minneapolis School of Anesthesia in 1969 (after about a month of classroom preparation), and I was eager to get started.

I could see a flurry of activity through the window in the door of OR four. When I entered I was stunned by the chaotic scene of a room full of people wearing bloody surgical garb. They were scrambling about, yelling out orders, rushing to cabinets and grabbing instruments for the surgical team—all of whom were bent over a patient whose pelvis and lower abdomen had been horribly ripped apart. Blood was dripping off the table and had even splattered on the walls. At one point I heard one of the surgeons say, "Damn, the whole right side of his pelvis is blown to bits."

Dr. Johnson noticed me. "Hi. I'm Norman Johnson. Squeeze the bag and keep pumping blood. There's a box of it right there, and I'll push the drugs. We're just giving this guy straight oxygen now, because he's basically moribund, and I'd be surprised if we get him off the table alive."

I gave him my name and immediately did as I was told. The patient had a big IV in each arm. It was all I could do to keep the units of blood pumping into each of them while squeezing the breathing bag. When I had finally collected myself, I asked Dr. Johnson what on earth had happened to the poor man. Johnson told me that the fellow owned a pawn shop in downtown Minneapolis and two guys had gone in to rob him that morning. According to his helper, who was currently in hiding, one of them had a revolver and the other a shotgun. As the owner was backing away from them, the one with the shotgun opened fire at close range, hitting him in the pelvis. Then they grabbed some jewelry and ran off. I was amazed that the man hadn't died on the spot after he was shot. It was a miracle that he made it to the hospital alive.

We had no modern-day monitors at the time—only a blood pressure cuff and precordial stethoscope. I could barely feel a weak carotid pulse on our patient and couldn't really say for sure we saw the needle on the blood pressure dial move at all. His pupils were fixed and dilated—not a good sign. Dr. Johnson kept pushing incremental doses of epinephrine into his IV, and I must have pumped at least fifteen units of blood into him. The surgical team worked feverishly; it seemed they were sucking out blood as fast as I was pumping it in. Finally, after about two hours of this, the man's head turned purple and mottled and he had no pulse. What an ignoble way to die.

This was the first time I had ever seen or been directly involved in such a grisly major trauma event. It bothered me that the poor man died, especially under those circumstances, but I was drawn to the prospect of being involved in more situations like this one—where I could have a significant role in possibly saving a life.

Those feelings stayed with me for the rest of my career.

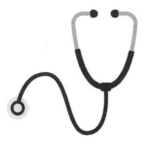

2. The ACDF

One morning in 2001, my first case of the day was scheduled as an anterior cervical discectomy and fusion (ACDF)—basically a neurosurgical case on the portion of the spine in a patient's neck. The approach is from the front, with the patient lying supine, and is done to remove a damaged intervertebral disc thereby relieving spinal cord or nerve root pressure and alleviate any corresponding pain, weakness, numbness, or tingling. Inasmuch as the surgery is close to the patient's face and in an area next to airway structures, intubation is necessary for the procedure.

My patient that morning was a middle-aged, otherwise healthy man who had undergone previous surgery without any problems. After introducing myself in the preop department, I had him open his mouth wide to inspect his airway. Immediately I was concerned about getting an endotracheal tube into his trachea because I could barely see the back of his throat. This was before the days of fiber-optic laryngoscopes and an airway like his could be a real problem. We had a difficult airway cart in the department which contained laryngoscope blades, mouthpieces, and a number of different stylets designed to fit inside endotracheal tubes which allow them to be bent in obtuse ways. I had the cart in the room all ready to go.

When the patient was on the OR table with all the anesthesia monitors hooked up, I called my attending MDA (medical doctor anesthesiologist) to come help me get the case started. After he arrived, I injected the IV drugs to anesthetize our patient, and after he was asleep I had a look in his mouth with a laryngoscope. All I could see in his throat was the very tip of the epiglottis—a flap of cartilage in the throat behind the tongue and on top of the larynx that folds down when you swallow to prevent food or liquids from entering your trachea. Without an adequate view of our patient's glottic opening into his trachea, I knew intubating him would be difficult.

I put a flexible stylet in the endotracheal tube, bent it into a curve, and tried slipping it under the epiglottis into where I thought his airway was. After several unsuccessful attempts, I let my attending MDA give it a try. He also bent the stylet different ways but couldn't get it into the trachea. I had a trick that I used for problems like this when I was working all alone in Bemidji, Minnesota called blind nasal intubation. The technique involves spraying the inside of one of the patient's nostrils with Neo-Synephrine to constrict blood vessels and keep them from bleeding, lubricating an endotracheal tube well with xylocaine jelly, and slowly inserting the tube through his sprayed nostril and down the throat toward the glottic opening, hoping it will drop into his airway. There's a chance the tube might go into the esophagus, but if that happens, pulling the tube back and lifting the patient's head up a bit while turning it slightly from side to side as you reinsert the tube should eventually work it into the patient's trachea.

It worked every time when I was all alone in Minnesota and had a problem like this, and if the patient had a full stomach, you could even do it while they were awake if you gave them light sedation and lubricated the endotracheal tube extremely well with xylocaine jelly. That would keep their airway reflexes intact in the event their stomach contents started to come up. I told the MDA about my experiences with that technique and suggested that he let me try it since I knew I could intubate our patient that way. I'm not sure if false pride or pure stubbornness was his problem, but he replied with a gruff "No."

Meanwhile, the neurosurgeon, who was also in the room waiting to get the case started, had watched our unsuccessful efforts at intubation and heard me tell the MDA about my blind nasal technique and the MDA's subsequent surly response. So, while the MDA had his back to me and was rummaging around in the difficult airway cart for something, the neurosurgeon motioned for me to go ahead with my idea. I thought to myself, *Well, it's his patient. If he wants me to do it, he's the ultimate authority on what happens in this OR and outranks the MDA.* So I quickly sprayed the patient's nostril, lubed the endotracheal tube, and slowly advanced it into the patient's nostril. As luck would have it, the tube dropped right into the patient's trachea on the first pass! When the MDA turned around and saw what had happened, he threw down the stylets he was holding and stomped out of the room with a scowl. Everybody had a good laugh after that. The neurosurgeon commented, "That was a pretty good example of how experience trumps book learning every time. He should've thanked you. He could've learned something."

The rest of the case went well. After I took my patient to the recovery room I expected I might hear something from the MDA whom I had just upstaged and basically proceeded against his wishes. I made a point of being in the office alone with him a few times so he'd have a chance to chew me out, but he never said a word. He used good judgment in that regard too, because I had a speech ready to go about how unappreciative he was and what's best for the patient didn't seem to be foremost in his mind.

Addendum:

Generally speaking, most oral surgery cases require the use of a nasotracheal tube with few exceptions. It's essential to become adept in nasal intubation. As I described in the prior episode, spraying the nose with Neo-Synephrine first and lubricating the nasotracheal tube well with xylocaine jelly is extremely important. I learned how to do nasal intubations in anesthesia school, but with the exception of one case, all the patients were under general anesthesia first, which made it pretty easy. In the '60s and '70s, fiber-optic indirect laryngoscopes hadn't been invented yet, making it crucial to become proficient at the blind nasotracheal intubation technique for difficult airways and patients with full stomachs. For every nasal intubation I performed during anesthesia school after the patient was anesthetized, I tried the blind technique first. The one awake blind nasal intubation I performed in school with the help of a staff CRNA was perfection; the nasotracheal tube dropped right into the trachea on the first try without any head manipulation. By the end of the program I was quite confident I wouldn't ever have a problem with it.

One Saturday evening in the '70s, I was called into our little northern Minnesota hospital for a case on a fellow who had been hit by a car. He had just finished dinner and was crossing the street to get to his car when the accident happened. The only injury he sustained was a compound fracture of his right femur. He was a big, relatively healthy guy. When I examined his airway, I noticed he had a large tongue, teeth in marginal-to-poor condition, and I could barely see the back of his throat. I didn't dare anesthetize him before trying to get an oral endotracheal tube into his trachea because of his very full stomach and apparent difficult airway. Due to increased gastric pressure, his partially digested dinner was sure to come up the minute he was anesthetized and would almost surely get into his lungs, causing all kinds of problems. After my assessment of his airway, I concluded that an oral intubation—even using the rapid sequence induction of anesthesia technique—was out of the question. My only option was to try an awake blind nasal intubation. I was nervous, to say the least.

I collected myself, put on my most confident demeanor, and explained everything to the patient. He understood the situation and was very cooperative. I didn't tell him that I'd only done one of these before while still in school. I also didn't mention that to the surgeon or staff.

After the patient was on the OR table, I lifted the back of it so that he was sitting up at a 30-degree angle. I gave him a very small dose of tranquilizer and sprayed one of his nostrils with Neo-Synephrine. I also sprayed his tongue and back of his throat, using an atomizer with 4 percent lidocaine, to minimize any irritation he might have as the nasotracheal tube slid through that area. Next, I lubricated the tube well with lidocaine jelly and gently inserted it into his nostril. I advanced it slowly and it slid in without resistance. He was tolerating the procedure very well. When I had him open his mouth, I could see the tip of the endotracheal tube in the back of his throat. Then, I put my ear close to my end of the tube so I could hear his breath sounds. As I slowly continued to advance it, the breath sounds became louder, until I felt his expired breath coming out of it on my ear. I kept advancing the tube until he coughed once, and a blast of air came rushing out of the tube, which indicated that it was most likely in his trachea. I inflated the cuff on the end of it, attached the connecter of the nasotracheal tube to the breathing hoses in the circuit of my anesthesia machine, and—lo and behold—I had a secure, well-sealed airway. I quickly anesthetized him with a dose of IV pentothal and turned on the anesthetic gasses. Now the surgery could begin.

The full stomach/airway issue wasn't completely resolved, however. Another critical time in situations like this is during the emergence of anesthesia. An anesthetized patient's protective airway reflexes don't return after anesthesia until they're completely awake. If the patient's stomach is still full of undigested food, the possibility of them vomiting and aspirating it into their lung while they're emerging from the general anesthetic is a big risk. The only way to minimize that is to empty their stomach while they're asleep.

I got an Ewald gastric lavage tube, which is one centimeter in diameter, lubricated it, and slowly inserted it down my sleeping patient's esophagus and into his stomach. I hooked it up to suction, and over the course of the two-hour surgery, sucked all the food out of his stomach. It took about an hour and one half to get it all out. Occasionally the Ewald tube would get plugged and I'd have to remove it, irrigate the large chunks of food out, and reinsert it. When only small particles were coming back, I irrigated the stomach with warm saline until everything came back clear. Finally, I was satisfied that he would emerge from the anesthetic with an empty stomach. The case ended, and my patient woke up just fine. He complained of leg pain but didn't have the least bit of nausea.

It was my first solo emergency blind nasal intubation, and I was pretty proud of myself.

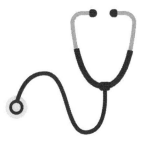

3. The Empty O2 Tank

In 1969 student CRNAs at a busy teaching hospital in downtown Minneapolis, were put in the call rotation just like regular staff. We always had a graduate CRNA on call with us but more often than not when there was a case to do we were eager to do it for the experience. The grads would let us go ahead without them, being only a phone call away if needed.

I had been in the program for about two months, and my first rotation was at the county hospital which received a lot of trauma and had a significant indigent patient census.

One day when I was on call, I had just worked about ten hours doing scheduled cases and was dead-tired. The call rooms were pretty Spartan, but they all had beds with clean sheets on them and when I got there I fell into a deep sleep almost immediately. About 2 a.m. my phone rang. It was the OR nurse telling me that we had a skin graft case to do right away. Hard to imagine that it needed to be done at that hour, but I headed over to the OR. When I arrived it turned out that an on-call intern and first-year medical student were going to do the case since that was the only time they could get on the schedule without much supervision. I, of course, had no say as to the timing of the case. I called my grad CRNA, who simply said, "Go ahead." The intern, medical student and I probably had no more than a year's experience between the three of us.

By today's standards of anesthesia practice, 1969 techniques were pretty crude. We didn't have a cardiac or oxygen saturation monitor, an anesthesia machine ventilator, an automatic blood pressure monitor, an electronic temperature monitor or any of the modern predictable anesthetic drugs we have today. Also, there was no pipeline oxygen or nitrous oxide in the room that we were going to do the case in, and all anesthetic gasses had to be delivered to the patient through a rudimentary anesthesia machine from two rows of four small tanks (four with oxygen and four with nitrous oxide) attached to the sides of the machine. Before anesthetizing any patient, it was essential to check all your equipment—especially the anesthesia machine. The machine had to be working perfectly, all the gasses flowing properly when the flow meters were turned on, all the fittings tight so that no leaks occurred between the patient and the machine while in use, and there had to be enough gas in the two rows of tanks to last for the whole case. Each anesthetic gas tank on the machine had to be turned on individually with the other ones tightly closed because the anesthesia machine was so old that it didn't have a check valve between them, which meant it was possible for the tanks to cross-fill.

I went through my pre-anesthetic checklist and everything was in order. I noticed that the machine had three full tanks of oxygen, three full tanks of nitrous oxide (laughing gas), and a half a tank of each.

The patient was a sixty-five-year-old alcoholic man in relatively poor physical health who had passed out in a drunken stupor with a cigarette in his hand and sustained second- and third-degree burns on his abdomen when his shirt caught fire. He'd been treated medically, and now it was time to graft those burns. I really didn't anticipate any instability issues with the patient because he'd been in the hospital for three weeks and was medically optimized. He was rather thin and had a slight expiratory wheeze from his years of smoking and associated mild COPD. Except for his bandaged abdomen he looked pretty good.

We placed the patient on the operating table and I got him hooked up to the few monitors I had. Next, I proceeded to have him breathe 100 percent oxygen for a few minutes before I administered sodium pentothal, followed by a muscle relaxant, until he became unconscious. I then placed a breathing tube into his windpipe through his mouth, secured it with tape to his upper lip and attached it to the breathing hoses from the anesthesia machine. I turned on the rest of the anesthetic gasses to mix with the oxygen he was already breathing, and we were all ready to start the case.

The dead tissue was going to have to be painstakingly removed bit by bit from the large burned areas on his abdomen, and then strips of normal skin tissue would be harvested from his thighs and grafted into place on his abdomen. My job was to keep him asleep for the whole procedure by administering the proper concentration of continuously flowing anesthetic gasses, mixed with oxygen, through his breathing tube and give occasional doses of intravenous sodium pentothal and muscle relaxant. All the while I had to squeeze the breathing bag on the anesthesia machine in a regular cadence to ventilate him.

As mentioned, it was 2 a.m. when I got called. By the time we got the case started it was 3 a.m. The room was warm, there was no music in the background, and I didn't know either of the fellows operating or the circulating nurse very well so there was no extraneous conversation in the room. The case dragged on and on, and I was fighting to stay awake.

At some point during the case, in the recesses of my mind, I vaguely heard a voice say, "That blood's awful dark isn't it?" Suddenly wide awake, I popped out of my chair like a jack-in-the-box and looked over the drapes at the surgical field. There, in the areas of his abdomen where they were removing dead skin, were oozing pools of dark-purple blood. I was horrified. The only way that can happen is if the patient isn't receiving enough oxygen in his ventilation, and I was in charge of that. Immediately, I looked at the oxygen flow meter on my anesthesia machine and was shocked to see that it was off. No oxygen was flowing at all. The only gas flowing was nitrous oxide. So, in effect, that's all I had been giving the patient for Heaven knows how long. I then saw that the small oxygen tank I had been using had run completely dry and was empty.

Immediately I cracked open a full oxygen tank on the machine, shut off the nitrous oxide, and proceeded to ventilate my patient as fast and with as large a breath of O2 as I could. I was so nervous and scared that I couldn't speak. My hands were shaking so much that I had to use them both to hold the breathing bag on my machine. Every bad outcome possible for the patient flashed through my mind, from severe brain damage to cardiac arrest. I thought, *Dear Lord, please let this man wake up and be just fine, and I promise I'll never go to sleep in the middle of a case again.* After about two minutes—which seemed like two hours—the blood on the surgical field started pinking up to the point that it began to look normal. I was only slightly relieved, however. His circulation had returned to normal, but his brain still could've had irreversible changes from oxygen deprivation, and he could wake up a veritable vegetable. The case was far from done, because of the lack of experience between the two operators, and I had only one thought in my mind: *Will he wake up and be normal?*

As I look back on my career, this was probably the most frightened I've ever been during a case. If I had caused the patient to have irreversible brain damage, it would have been my last day in the program—to say nothing of having it on my conscience forever. Whatever damage I may have caused was already done, and the waiting for this case to be finished was awful. To add to my misery, I had to appear outwardly calm so that no one else in the room would be rattled by my inner turmoil. Bear in mind that I was only twenty-seven years old and had never dealt with stress of this intensity in my life.

The case inched along at a snail's pace, as my anxiety mounted. Finally, at about 7:30 a.m., it finished and it was time for my patient to wake up. I turned all the anesthetic gasses off and let the man start breathing 100 percent oxygen spontaneously. A good sign, because at least that showed that the respiratory center in his brain was still working. I had given him some narcotics intravenously way back at the start of the case, which can sometimes cause a slow emergence from anesthesia, but in this case he started to move his extremities and groan. I called his name, and he opened his eyes. I was ecstatic! Next, I told him to take a deep breath and wiggle his toes, both of which he did. I asked him if he knew where he was, and he answered that he was in the hospital in surgery having skin grafts. He also knew what year it was and that Nixon was president.

I had dodged a bullet. The relief I experienced at that moment is probably akin to what people who've had a near-death experience and survived unscathed go through. I took my patient to the recovery room, gave the nurse report, and went to the break room, exhausted. Nobody ever asked me about the case or why the blood was dark for that brief period during the procedure so I never told anyone about it.

I learned a valuable lesson that day and in all the rest of my years in anesthesia, I've never fallen asleep during a case again.

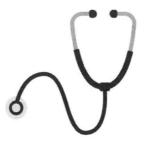

4. The Ladies' Man

We were finishing up an appendectomy around 1:30 in the morning one Saturday in November when a call came through from the emergency room. We were told a gunshot injury was coming in from a small town just north of Bemidji. It was deer hunting season then and not unusual to get an occasional hunting accident, since the woods around town were full of hunters from all over the state. All of them carried high-powered rifles, and quite a few weren't there to hunt as much as party down.

The surgeon and I finished up our case and went down to the ER to wait. After about thirty minutes, the ambulance arrived and pulled into the ER portico. The driver told us it had happened in the liquor store and that our patient was still pretty drunk but somewhat coherent. We opened the back doors of the ambulance to an overwhelming odor of whiskey, vomit, and feces. There laying on the gurney was a large man still in his blaze-orange hunting suit with a pile of bloody bath towels stuffed between his legs. We crawled into the ambulance and the surgeon put on gloves to lift up the towels and see what was underneath.

As he did, the patient said, "Do a good job, doc. I'm quite a ladies' man, you know." The surgeon lifted the towels and in the patient's crotch where his genitals should be was a huge, gaping, oozing sore with absolutely no remnants left of them whatsoever.

The surgeon said, "You mean, you *were* quite a ladies' man!"

His hunting suit in the area around the wound was full of powder burns so obviously he had been shot point-blank. The driver told us that the guy had been in the liquor store drinking for quite a while and flirting with/chasing after one of the ladies from the nearby reservation. She evidently got tired of his advances, picked up a nearby 20-gauge shotgun loaded with a slug, and shot him in the crotch.

We took the fellow into the ER and got him stripped and his crotch packed and prepped for surgery. Once he was in the operating room and asleep, the surgeon cleaned up his wound, cut away all the dead tissue, stopped the bleeding, and irrigated it with antibiotics. It was impossible to close that gaping crater so it was packed with sterile dressings. The circulator called Minneapolis to send their air ambulance and come take our fellow home the next morning.

I often wondered when he arrived home how he explained to his family how he had lost all his manhood.

To my knowledge, no one was ever charged with a crime.

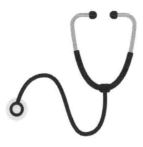

5. The White Mustang

One fall in the 1970s, I went archery elk hunting for a week in Colorado with two friends, one of whom was a veterinarian. We drove out in his practice wagon—a big Chevrolet Carryall equipped with all his medical supplies and tools of the trade for country calls, with plenty of room left over for our hunting gear. Our route took us from northern Minnesota through the Wyoming mountains and down into Colorado. We drove straight through both ways with one of us sleeping and the other two driving and navigating.

Early one morning we were driving on a mile-high, two-lane winding mountain road near Lusk, Wyoming and just chugging along because of the thin mountain air and the Chevy having a Minnesota-tuned carburetor. At one point a white Ford Mustang pulled up behind us and, because of the road, couldn't pass us and there was no shoulder we could pull over on to let him by. He was behind us for quite a few miles until finally the road straightened out a bit and he went whizzing by. I was driving at the time and noticed as the Mustang passed that there were a couple of young boys in the front seat. They sped off, and we just kept chugging along.

A mile further on, the mountain opened up away from the road, leading into a large grassy area on our left. As we came upon it we noticed the white Mustang about thirty yards off into the grass, upside down, doors open and the two boys lying on the ground nearby about thirty feet apart. We immediately pulled off the road and ran over. One of the boys was screaming loudly about his back hurting and the other lay motionless, his skin mottled purple and making respiratory efforts but obviously had an airway obstruction. I told my friend, an ex-Vietnam Army corpsman, to go check the boy who was screaming while my veterinarian friend and I rushed over to the unconscious boy. He was completely flaccid, his head flexed forward and not moving any air. I didn't want to move his head for fear he might have an unstable neck injury, so I had my friend hold his head steady while I managed to reach a gloved hand into his mouth and pull his tongue forward.

I heard the boy gasp a little, so I had my veterinarian friend run back to his practice wagon to get me whatever animal airway device he might have to hold this kid's mouth open and tongue in place. He brought me a wedge that he used to hold dogs' mouths open, which worked perfectly. I stuck it between the boy's teeth, on one side of his mouth, and pulled his tongue way out. Right away, he started taking huge breaths. Almost immediately his color improved and, much to our delight, he started moving all his extremities. Within minutes he opened his eyes and tried to sit up but held him down, telling him not to move much until he was wide awake. I ran through a few quick battlefield-type neurology checks, all of which he passed with flying colors. He appeared to have just been knocked out.

My veterinarian friend went to his Carryall to see if he could raise somebody in the area on his CB radio that could send an ambulance. It took him the better part of fifteen minutes to get any kind of response and when he did, thankfully, it was the sheriff. About a half hour later, the sheriff and an ambulance showed up. I identified myself, gave the EMTs a quick report on the boys, and went to tell the sheriff what had happened. He was a tall, muscular guy—the stereotypical good-looking lawman you see in every Hollywood movie. He wore dark aviator sunglasses, a large Stetson cowboy hat, and had a big .44 on his hip.

He said to me, "Y'all done a damn fine job here boys and these young whelps oughtta be real thankful you come along. That'n there woulda been a goner fer sure. Looks like you gotta a fair piece of huntin' to do. So, you kin' go now and, we'll take 'er from here." He never asked our names, where we were from, or anything about us so we all thanked him and left.

The sheriff was right: The unconscious kid would've died for sure. It must have been Divine intervention that we showed up with the expertise to save him.

We chuckled over the sheriff's comments for the rest of the trip.

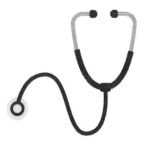

6. The Back Booth

On a cold, snowy evening in January, as we were doing a late case, a call came into the operating room from the owner of a beer tavern downtown. He wondered if our surgeon could come by the bar when he was done working and check out a patron he was worried about. The surgeon said he'd be glad to as soon as he finished the case. I told him he wasn't going to check somebody in a bar at this time of night without me, so after the case off we went.

The tavern was in the middle of downtown Bemidji, and because of the weather and the hour, nobody was out on the streets. We walked into the place and were greeted by the owner from behind the bar. He gestured toward the back, where a row of booths stood, telling us that the fellow was in the last booth on the right. When we got there, we found a thin, older man sitting upright and leaning against the back of the booth and the wall. His arms were on the table, his eyes closed, his head was cocked over to the left and a half-full glass of beer sat in front of him. He was not breathing, his face was a deep grayish-purple and he was quite obviously dead. The doctor and I both felt for a carotid or radial pulse and, of course, there was none. When we returned to the owner and announced our findings, he slapped his hand on the bar and announced loudly, "I thought so. He hasn't ordered a beer in over an hour."

I couldn't stand it and burst out laughing.

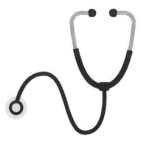

7. Poor Bob

I was called to obstetrics one afternoon to perform an epidural anesthetic on a patient in labor. To accomplish this, a catheter is threaded into a small space (epidural space) in the patient's back between their vertebrae and adjacent to the spinal canal, using sterile technique. The catheter is then hooked to a line attached to a bag of local anesthetic mixture in a digital pump. The pump slowly meters that mixture into the epidural space and should significantly dull or take away all the pain of uterine contractions. Correctly placed, it can be left in place for several days.

To accomplish this procedure, I would usually have my patient sit up on the edge of the bed facing her husband and she'd put her arms around him with her head bent forward, resting on his shoulder while he kept his arms around her. This way, he could keep a good hold on her during the procedure so she wouldn't move much during uterine contractions while I was working.

My patient was a young woman in advanced labor experiencing her first childbirth and complaining loudly with each contraction. She was in a birthing room with her husband who was looking rather bewildered while trying to comfort her.

After she was in position, I went behind her and had her round her back out as much as possible toward me to open up the spaces between her vertebrae so I could find my landmarks. As I was washing her back with my sterilizing prep solution, I noticed that she was leaning about ten degrees to the right instead of sitting straight up, so I asked her husband to please move her a little more to the left.

He did so and asked, "Like this?"

When the patient heard her husband, she said in a loud voice right into his ear, "Bob, shut up!"

He replied, "But honey, I was just answering Ron."

She yelled, "Bob, I said *shut the f*ck up!*"

This outburst really made me mad, and I told her, "That's enough of this kind of talk and the epidural is not going into your back if I hear any more of it. You can just labor the old-fashioned way—all natural!"

Her answer was, "Well, okay. He can talk to you, but *nobody the f*ck else!*"

I looked at Bob, whose face was quivering and bright red as he struggled for control. I thought to myself, what a witch. *Poor Bob. I bet that's not the first time she's talked to him like that.* The rest of the procedure went very well and the epidural gave her excellent labor pain relief, but she never acknowledged to me or Bob any kind of gratitude for our efforts.

I laughed all the way back to the anesthesia department, while thinking to myself, *Poor Bob!*

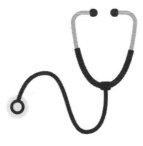

8. The Bet

On a winter morning in 1973, my first case of the day was a cesarean section on a healthy twenty-nine-year-old lady. The obstetrician preferred using general anesthesia on these cases as opposed to a regional spinal or epidural. The technique was to put the patient on the operating table, get her IV started and a liter of IV fluid into her while they were prepping and draping her belly, and have the surgical team gowned and gloved and standing by all ready to go. Once the patient was prepped, I'd give her a dose of sodium pentothal and quick-acting muscle relaxant and as soon as she closed her eyes and was unconscious, I'd give them the okay to start.

Our thinking was that if the baby was out quickly (say, under a minute) the pentothal wouldn't have enough circulation time in the mother to cross the placental barrier and get to the baby, causing the newborn to be anesthetized too. As soon as the umbilical cord was clamped, I would turn on anesthetic gasses and put the mother deeply asleep. I discussed all of this with our patient, and she was fine with it.

One caveat to this particular case was that the patient's husband had wagered five thousand dollars that the baby was going to be born a boy. She told me that in preop, saying that she wished he hadn't and that they didn't have that kind of money to risk.

After she was all prepped and draped, I gave her the pentothal and muscle relaxant and as I was putting in her breathing tube I told the team to go ahead. Her doctor made the incision, and in less than a minute had the baby out—a beautiful little girl. I looked up and burst out laughing saying, "Good. I'm glad that son of a bitch lost his money." I turned on the anesthetic gasses, and everybody laughed. Our cute little newborn girl went off to the nursery, and in about forty-five minutes the case was over, and the dressings were on.

I let the patient wake up, and as I was taking her to the recovery room, I called to her softly, telling her that she had a beautiful baby girl. When we arrived at the recovery room she was fully awake. She looked at me and said, "Can I ask you a question?" I said, "Of course, you may," whereupon she asked, "Who was it that called my husband a son of a bitch?" That really surprised me!

After the small induction dose of Pentothal I'd given her, the surgeon had started the procedure immediately. Evidently the dose hadn't circulated to her brain sufficiently to render her completely unconscious and she heard my comment. I stuttered and stammered a bit, then finally said, "Well, I'm sorry to say I was the one who said it." She got a strange look on her face and said, "Well, he is a son of a bitch. We don't have five thousand dollars to spare, damn him."

What a relief! I was like a man out of prison, having already envisioned explaining myself to the hospital administrator and maybe even the board of directors—to say nothing of what might have happened had word of the incident gotten out into the community.

I learned a very valuable lesson that day about conversations and comments around chemically altered patients. I never had that problem again.

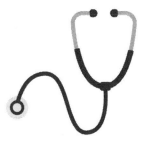

9. Two Interesting Patients

While working in a relatively small hospital in Dunedin, Florida in 1989, a pacemaker insertion case was added to the late-afternoon schedule in my room. I got set up for it and went to preop to see my patient. He was an alert and well-oriented eighty-nine-year-old man with a very slow heart rate. After looking his chart over and introducing myself, I went through the perfunctory pre-pacemaker conversation with him and he understood everything to my satisfaction. The man had a heavy German accent, so I asked him how long he had been in this country. He said that he had come here in the early 1950s after the war and had been an American citizen since the '60s. I then posed the same question I usually ask all old German immigrants who spent World War II in Europe: "Did you ever see der Fuhrer?"

He answered me with such a heavy accent that I didn't quite understand, so I repeated the question. He said, "I was one of his interpreters." That gave me goose bumps. I asked him what Hitler was like. He said, "Well, I was only one of his interpreters, and mostly I was with him at his residences. And we—his house staff—knew what a monster he was and what a terrible temper he had, because we'd seen him screaming at his general staff. But to us, a kinder, nicer, and more generous man you've never met. He didn't smoke or drink, he was a vegetarian, and he loved animals. He doted on his German shepherd, Blondi." That really surprised me. I wanted to pursue our conversation further, but we had only a short time together due to his heart condition and the need to get his pacemaker implanted.

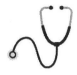

The first patient I attended to one morning in the mid-1990s was an old fellow who needed minor surgery. After perusing his chart, I introduced myself and went through my usual routine, discussing where he was originally from, what kind of work he did, etc. He happened to be a retired Navy veteran and told me about the time he served as an officer on a light cruiser, which happened to be the first ship to enter the Nagasaki harbor on a fact-finding mission after the atomic bomb was dropped there during World War II. He said a four thousand-foot mountain, with a Mitsubishi armament manufacturing plant built into it, had been constructed by the harbor for protection. When his ship entered the harbor he noticed that the mountain was gone, completely flattened. He said that picture of devastation will be in his mind forever.

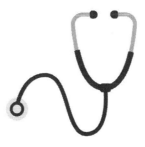

10. Two Neurosurgery Stories

One morning I was working with Kevin on a complicated brain tumor case. We had our middle-aged male patient anesthetized and lying supine, propped up at a ten-degree angle. His head was stabilized by special cranial tongs called a Mayfield head holder which attached to the OR table. The tongs circled one half of his head and were held in place by short, sharp spikes. The patient was relatively healthy, and the case progressed quite nicely. Kevin had his craniotomy incision (opening into the skull) on the top of the man's head and was reaching into it with instruments to resect the tumor. As I watched him work, I noticed that when he inserted an instrument it seemed to sink three to four inches into the patient's brain. Finally, I said to him, "For god's sake, Kevin. Where the hell are you putting that forceps?" Without missing a beat, he responded, "Right next to his soul!" That gave me a chill. For the rest of my career, I thought of that statement every time I had a craniotomy case.

Brain aneurysms are very serious, and the surgery to fix them is delicate and complicated. They present a lot of issues and concerns for both anesthesia and the surgical team, as you might imagine.

Kevin Sweeney and I were about two hours into such a case on a middle-aged lady one morning back in the early '90s. Everything was going well, and the patient was stable under anesthesia. In order to reach the aneurysm, Kevin had to do a very delicate and time-consuming dissection. He had to separate brain tissues to adequately expose the aneurysm and apply a special clip to it to prevent it from rupturing. Pressure on the aneurysm from surrounding brain tissue is often the main factor keeping it from rupturing spontaneously and abruptly relieving that pressure can trigger a massive bleed.

As Kevin got down to the aneurysm, he alerted the team so we could prepare for all possibilities. When we were ready, he loaded the aneurysm clip into its holder in his right hand, and with his left hand very gingerly, deftly and delicately retracted the last small portion of the brain covering it. Immediately a sudden gush of blood filled the incision and spilled over onto the floor! Without a moment's hesitation Kevin thrust the clip into that pool and applied the clip blindly. Miraculously, the bleeding stopped, and when he suctioned out the residual blood, the clip had been applied to the aneurysm perfectly. His only comment afterward was, "It's like doing surgery in an inkwell." *(Good line.)*

The patient woke up well, with all her neurological parameters intact and we took her to the recovery room and later to ICU.

In all my years in the anesthesia business, I've never witnessed anything as dramatic as what Kevin Sweeney did that day. His extensive training and fearlessness saved that lady's life.

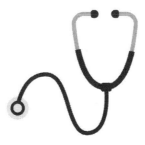

11. Three Tattoo Stories

Our anesthesia group in St. Petersburg, Florida also covered three surgicenters where I frequently worked. The patients at these places were usually healthy and in for minor surgeries. My first case one morning was on a thirtyish young woman with a cyst on her back. For the surgeon to remove it, she would need to be turned over and positioned on her stomach after she was asleep. I entered her cubicle, perused her chart, and introduced myself.

"Good morning. I'm Ron Whitchurch from the anesthesia department, and I'll be putting you to sleep today for the doctor to remove that cyst on your back." I said.

She replied, "Oh, so you're Ron! You know what? I have your name tattooed on my ass." That surprised me, so I asked her to please let me see it. "Oh, no," she replied. "You'll have plenty of time to see it after I'm asleep and turned over."

Now I was focused, thinking that I didn't even know this woman. How could my name be there? I asked her if she was pulling my leg, and she replied with a straight face, "No way. You'll see I'm not lying. Your name is tattooed on my ass in big letters, and it's impressive."

When it came time to bring her to the operating room and start the case, I put her to sleep on the gurney so we could turn her over to the OR table. After she was positioned on her belly, the circulating nurse pulled her gown aside—and there it was, across her right buttock in large, beautiful script lettering. A tattoo that read, "YOUR NAME." The whole room roared with laughter at it and me for being so completely taken in by her story.

I realized that this was too good an opportunity to miss, so I told the circulator to cover it up and call my attending anesthesiologist into the room. He came in, questioning whether anything was wrong. I told him no but that I thought we had one of his old girlfriends here on the table. He got a concerned, perplexed look on his face. Then, he looked at her name band and said he didn't know the girl at all. I said, "Come clean now, Dwight. That's very surprising, because it's definitely your name tattooed on her ass." Meanwhile, the staff was chortling to themselves.

Now he had a horrified look on his face and argued, "She does not. You're shitting me."

I said, "Okay. If that's what you think, come have a look."

The circulating nurse pulled her gown back to show him the tattoo, and I've never seen anyone laugh harder than he did that day. He even had to go over and sit on a stool—that's how hard he was laughing. We tried to pull it on the surgeon too, but he'd already heard about it.

It was one of the most enjoyable spoofs I've ever experienced in all my years in the OR, and I chuckle about it to this day. I bet the lady is still having fun with that ruse.

One day, while getting an elderly lady on the OR table ready to go to sleep and hooking up all the monitors, I noticed a pretty flower tattoo up by her shoulder as I was applying the EKG stickers to her chest. I said, "That's a pretty rose you have tattooed there." She retorted, "What's the matter with you? That's a coiled-up snake. Can't you tell?" The OR folks laughed about that for the rest of the day. I shouldn't have said anything, because her skin was wrinkled, and I really couldn't tell for sure what it was.

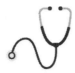

One of my many patients happened to be a middle-aged, muscular fellow covered in tattoos from head to foot. Only his face and hands were devoid of ink. He told me he started getting them in the service and just kept adding more after his discharge, but now there wasn't any space left. They were all well done and very colorful. I asked him if he had any tattoos where nobody could see them and he folded down his bottom lip, like a pout, in response. On the inside of it, tattooed on the mucous membrane in big block letters so that I could clearly read them, were the words: "F*CK YOU." He told me that it was the perfect comeback for whenever he was at a party and somebody who was "full of shit" tried to tell him something. All he had to do was flip his lip at them, and they usually shut up and walked away. I asked him if that one had hurt when it was done, and he said, "Nah. I was drunk as hell at the time."

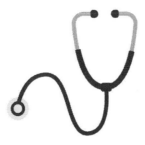

12. The Diamond Ring

In Bemidji, we frequently had children come to the OR for various surgeries such as tonsillectomies, hernia repairs, crossed eyes, injuries, etc. The kids between about five and ten years old were always frightened, so I'd tell them they just had to blow up a balloon to go to sleep. If they'd allow me to put an IV in them, we'd have a lot of fun. After they were on the OR table with their IV running, and I was all set to go, I'd ask if they wanted to play a little game with me and invariably, they said yes.

If a little boy was the one on the table, I'd tell him, "Okay, now here's the deal. If you had a choice, what would you rather have: a minibike or a brand new .22 rifle?" If it was a little girl, I'd have her choose between a diamond ring or fur coat. Those choices excited them, and after they picked their prize, I'd tell them the rules: If they could count from one all the way to ten before they went to sleep, they'd win the prize. The catch was that they couldn't start counting until I told them to. When the team was in the room and all ready to go, I'd inject a dose of pentothal into their IV and wait until I saw that they were starting to get a little bit sleepy. Then, I'd tell them to start counting. Usually, they didn't make it past three, but occasionally one would get all the way to five. This was so much fun that I played it with the kids for years—that is, until the day a surgeon ruined it.

I had a cute little nine-year-old girl as a patient for an abdominal scar revision from an old farm injury. She had a sweet personality and was very compliant with everything, even allowing me to start her IV. When she was on the OR table and the team was all in place, just before we were ready to get started, I asked her if she wanted to play the aforementioned game, and she jumped at the chance. I explained the rules, and she chose the diamond ring. The surgeon was standing right next to us at the table, and as I picked up the pentothal syringe, he blurted out, "Okay, start counting." I wasn't even close to ready for her to do that! I hustled to get my pentothal plugged into the IV line, but she was already up to six. I gave her an induction dose, but it was too late. "Nine…," she counted. "Ten, eleven, twelve, thhhhirteeeee…" The surgeon laughed like crazy, along with everybody else—except me. I told him that I hoped she didn't remember getting to thirteen, because if so, he could buy her the diamond ring.

The case went uneventfully, and in the recovery room I cautioned everybody to please not bring up the diamond ring contest.

The next day, I happened to run into my surgeon friend downtown—the same one who told the little girl to start counting the day before, and he told me, "Ron, you've got a very unhappy little girl up on the third floor of the hospital that woke up yesterday and doesn't have a diamond ring."

I'd hoped she wouldn't remember it. My wife and I quickly headed over to Woolworths and bought the biggest diamond ring they had. It was a huge sparkler and we wrapped it up in fancy paper and headed over to the hospital. When we arrived at the cute little girl's room, she was so happy to see me. I'm sure she knew why I'd come. I went over, gave her a big hug, and showed her the pretty present I had for her. Her eyes lit up, and when she saw the diamond ring she let out a loud shriek. There has probably never been a happier little girl in the world than she was at that moment.

I told her she was the only one who ever won the prize, and now that we finally had a winner, I was going to end the contest, which I did. Lesson learned…

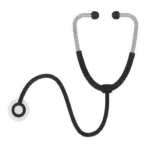

13. An Atheist

In 1972 I worked as a CRNA in Bemidji, Minnesota about three hundred miles north of Minneapolis. My mother was living in Minneapolis at the time and had just taken a job at a rather large congregational church in South Minneapolis. She was a religious educator, did her undergraduate work at Rockford College and post-graduate education at the University of Minnesota, and was the director of religious education at the church. After about six months in her new capacity, the church secretary put a little note about her in the Sunday services program. The secretary, a sweet retired Scandinavian lady, had interviewed my mother for about two hours to get the material for her synopsis.

I wish I still had a copy of the program, but in all my family's moves, I lost it. It went something like this:

Katherine Whitchurch is our new director of Christian education here at Plymouth. She has an extensive background in business and religious teaching. She was born and raised in Rockford, Illinois, and had all of her undergraduate college education at Rockford College, graduating with a bachelor's degree in education. She moved to Minneapolis in 1947 and in 1961 went back to graduate school at the University of Minnesota to obtain a master's degree in theology.

She has been the director of religious education at Lynnhurst Congregational Church, alumni director at Rockford College, and director of fundraising at the Minneapolis branch of the Boys Club of America, and now we welcome her as our new religious education director.

Except for the four-year period as alumni director, she has lived in Minneapolis continuously since 1947.

*She has one son, Ronald, who is an **Atheist** in Bemidji, MN.*

The sweet secretary may have misspelled anesthetist but my guess is that she only heard *atheist*. Either way, it was really funny. The best part is, not one person called to inquire about it, and no one in the congregation ever brought it up to my mother. They all must have thought, *Oh, that poor woman. How she must have suffered, having an atheist for a son.* When I attended church with her on our visits, not a word was ever spoken about it either. Everybody was exceptionally friendly—they probably thought she needed all the help she could get to show me the light.

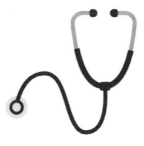

14. The Arm Block

Back in the mid-1970s, regional anesthesia for extremities was not as sophisticated as it is today. We didn't have portable ultrasound imaging or much of the equipment and drugs that are now in common use. In order to perform an axillary (armpit) block, which would effectively make the patient's whole arm numb, we had to really know our anatomy. An anesthesia practitioner would place the patient's arm over their head in order to palpate the armpit and feel for an axillary artery pulse. The axillary artery supplies blood to the lower arm, and the bundle of nerves for innervation and sensation of the arm runs through its sheath. Using sterile technique, local anesthetic can be injected into the sheath to block those nerves, thereby making the patient's arm completely numb. It's a valuable type of regional anesthesia that spares the patient a general anesthetic for lower arm surgery.

My first planned case one morning in February 1979 was to be a carpal tunnel release on a morbidly obese man, whom I'll call Kenny. Carpal tunnel surgery is performed on the wrist and is a soft tissue operation. It just so happened that I knew the fellow fairly well and had often thought how I would handle him if I ever got him as a patient. To complicate my anesthetic assessment, he had the type of jaw anatomy that would make it very difficult to control or support his airway once he was asleep so he was a perfect candidate for an axillary block. I discussed it with the surgeon, who agreed that we did not want to have to give this fellow a general anesthetic if we could avoid it. I spoke to the patient and his wife in preop and they were fine with the procedure.

When Kenny was on the OR table with his IV running, I gave him a light tranquilizer and small dose of short-acting narcotic. After he was pleasantly sedated, I lifted his arm over his head to find his axillary artery pulse. He was so obese and had such huge, flabby upper arms that even with his arm over his head it didn't expose the whole armpit, and when I reached in there to palpate the pulse, my hand disappeared to the wrist. It was all but impossible to feel an axillary pulse. I poked around, still unsure if I really felt anything. When I did, I wasn't sure whose pulse it was—mine or his. I had a fairly good idea of where the artery and nerve bundles were, so after about fifteen minutes of this, I decided to proceed and asked Kenny to please let me know the minute he felt anything, like an electric shock down his arm. I had the nurse get a good, two handed, grip on his arm.

When a patient feels a shock it can be a big surprise making them jump and pull their arm away. I wasn't prepared for what happened next. When I infiltrated a little local anesthetic in the skin to make it numb for the longer anesthetic needle to be inserted, he jerked his arm loose and let out a bloodcurdling scream. That startled me and the nurse—we both jumped back. I quickly got some more tranquilizer and narcotic into him and tried to calm him down a bit, explaining that was just a little skin-numbing medicine. He apologized and said he'd try to hold still. We got his arm up over his head again, and this time I wrapped it with two-inch tape and all around the OR table, in case we had a repeat performance. I infiltrated more local anesthetic into the already-numbed area, waited a few minutes, and then slowly inserted the longer anesthetic delivery needle in toward the axillary nerve bundle, reminding him to let me know if he felt any kind of electric shock.

Suddenly he let out another loud scream and yelled, "Oh, Ron! There, there, there. Ron, stop. Stop, stop, ouch, ow, ow, ow." I was ready for it this time. His arm didn't move, but he was doing a backbend on the table and kicking his legs. I had to get one of the orderlies to come and hold him down. I immediately stopped inserting the needle and asked him where he felt the electric shock. "All over my whole body," he replied. I was pretty sure that wasn't the case, so when he finally calmed down, I gingerly advanced my anesthetic needle forward. He let out another bloodcurdling scream and tried to grab me with his free arm, but the orderly grabbed it right away. I let him calm down again, told the nurse to give him a little more sedation, and very slowly and gingerly injected my anesthetic mixture into what I hoped was the axillary nerve sheath.

He was calm at that point because the mixture numbed the area as I injected it. By then about one hour had gone by, and everybody in the room, including me, was on edge. I told the surgeon that I wasn't at all confident my block was going to be effective because of Kenny's obesity and inability to cooperate. The surgeon said that he could infiltrate some local anesthetic in the operative site if necessary, and I could give him a little more sedation. By now everything I'd given Kenny in his IV had caught up to him, and he was pleasantly snoring. We got his operative arm scrubbed up with sterilizing prep solution, secured it to the table, and put the surgical drapes on.

I motioned for the surgeon to inject a little local into the operative site. The little prick of that local needle into his wrist woke him up, and he gave another loud shriek! That told us all we needed to know about my failed axillary block. I quickly gave him more sedation, consisting of incremental doses of sodium pentothal. It was just enough to put him in the twilight zone and lie still but not enough to make him stop breathing. The surgeon put more local in the operative site and proceeded with the surgery. Kenny would periodically wake up a little and moan, whereupon I'd dose him again, and he'd drift off. After about forty-five minutes, the surgery was finished, and we moved him to the recovery room.

After all the sedation I'd given Kenny, and because of how numb his operative field was from what the surgeon had injected, it took him a few hours to wake up. I hoped that all the medication I'd given him would provide a good measure of amnesia so he wouldn't be troubled by it and annoyed with me forever. He finally got dressed and went home.

Bemidji is a small, northern Minnesota town that is cold and bleak in the winter with many days of below-zero temperatures. The roads are slippery, it snows frequently, and the sky seems perpetually overcast and gray. Spring never really arrives until toward the end of May. In order to break up the weather-induced monotony, my wife and I would occasionally plan a getaway to either Minneapolis or Fargo, North Dakota.

One January in 1981 we planned a long weekend trip to the Fargo Holiday Inn and invited an old childhood friend and his wife from Minneapolis to join us. We met them on Saturday afternoon and decided to go to the inn's hot tub for a while to warm up and catch up. We were the only ones in the tub and enjoyed a few libations and conversation. After a half hour another couple headed over to the tub. When I saw who it was, I almost had an anxiety attack. It was none other than Kenny and his wife and he hadn't lost a bit of weight since our encounter in surgery.

I watched the pair climb into the hot tub and settle in directly opposite me. I was a little nervous, to say the least, and felt obliged to make some kind of conversation. "Hi, Kenny," I began. "How're you doing? I hope your wrist is okay. I really feel bad about all the trouble we had trying to numb up your arm and causing you pain back when we fixed it."

He replied, "Ron, put that out of your mind! Don't worry about it for a minute, because it was no problem at all. As a matter of fact, I'd forgotten all about it until you brought it up just now. It really was nothing and didn't bother me a bit."

I said, "Gee, thanks, Kenny, because I thought I must have really traumatized you. I appreciate you saying that."

After that exchange, we shared more light conversation, until my wife mentioned to me that it was time to get ready for dinner. Kenny was in a deep conversation with his wife, and I told our friends that we'd meet them later in the dining room.

My wife and I changed clothes and at the appointed time went to the dining room. When our friends arrived, the husband said to me, "What in the hell did you do to that fat guy that we met in the hot tub?"

I said, "Why do you ask?"

My friend replied, "You should have heard what he said about you after you left. Obviously he didn't know that we were together, and he told his wife in a rather loud voice, 'That son of a bitch Ron damn near killed me. He had about a foot-long needle that he kept stabbing into my armpit, and it hurt like hell, and the more I screamed the harder he did it. He finally quit, but if he hadn't, I'd have probably punched the asshole.'"

That was quite a surprise and I told him all about the ordeal I'd put Kenny through trying to make his arm numb. We all had a good laugh over it. To this day, I can still see that scene in my mind.

I think every practitioner wonders what their patients truly think of them after the fact. These days, almost everyone gets a survey from their healthcare facility relatively soon after their visit. Back in the old days there was nothing like that, and in our little town you were more apt to hear about your experience with a patient through the grapevine. I can only wonder how many people in town heard Kenny's story.

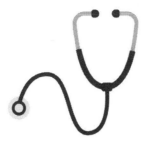

15. The Hiccups

In 1970 I was a senior student at the Minneapolis School of Anesthesia. For our clinical experiences, we rotated between five hospitals in the Minneapolis area, which gave us quite a well-rounded exposure to a variety of anesthesia techniques.

A patient hiccupping while under anesthesia—especially on an abdominal case—is a real problem. It completely disrupts the operative field. The anesthetic agents in use then weren't as sophisticated as they are now, and hiccups were not uncommon and every practitioner had their own method of treating them.

One morning, in the middle of a rather lengthy upper abdominal case, my patient developed a bad case of hiccups and about every ten seconds his abdominal contents would jump up through the incision. I tried everything I could think of, from suctioning his throat to giving him large inspiratory and slightly prolonged breaths, all to no avail. The surgeon couldn't proceed under those circumstances, so I called for my attending anesthesiologist. After I explained everything, he said to me, "Ronald, it's good that you called me. I have a surefire way to cure these, which I'm very surprised they haven't taught you in school. It's Ritalin, my boy. Get me a vial of that, and I'll show you how it works."

I had my circulating nurse get me a couple of vials right away. My attending snatched one of them up, drew up a syringe full, and injected it into the patient's IV, whereupon the hiccups magically stopped. We were all amazed! My doctor turned to me and said, "You see what I mean, Ronald? This stuff is a miracle drug for hiccups. I don't know why they don't teach all of you this.

I'm going to have to speak to the director about that. Now, when you go back to class, be sure to share this with everybody. It's a valuable addition to our anesthesia armamentarium, and they all need to know about it." I, of course, dutifully said that I certainly would. He left the room, and we got the case underway again.

Injectable Ritalin is supplied with two vials: one is Ritalin powder, and the other is saline diluent that must be mixed with the powder to put it into solution before administration. When I looked at the anesthesia cart I saw the two vials my attending had just used, but one still had powder in it. In his haste to get the hiccups cured and show me his expertise, he hadn't taken the time to mix up the Ritalin and had only injected the saline diluent. In essence, the hiccups had cured themselves. I chuckled to myself for the rest of the case over that, though I didn't dare mention it to him and burst his bubble. When I got to class later I heeded his advice and shared it with everybody, to gales of laughter.

I never called for Ritalin again in all my years of work.

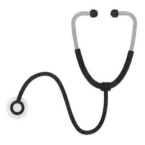

16. The Elevator

I was nearing the end of my senior year in anesthesia school and rotating through a hospital in St. Louis Park, Minnesota, when the chief of anesthesia came to me one morning and said, "Ron, I just got a call from ICU. There's a patient up there that needs to be intubated. You're far enough along in the program, and I've watched you, so go up there by yourself and take care of it. You don't need any help. And by the way, you don't have to hurry because the patient's airway isn't obstructed. He's just getting worn out from struggling to breathe because of his COPD."

Intubation consists of placing a breathing tube through the patient's mouth and into their trachea with the use of a lighted device called a laryngoscope. The breathing tube is secured in place with tape and then usually hooked up to a ventilator.

I got my lab coat on, name badge clearly identifying me as a member of the anesthesia department, and went to the elevator. The ICU was several floors above us and when the elevator arrived, four people were already inside. I stepped in and immediately noticed an awful, almost overpowering odor of nasty, fetid flatulence in the air. Because I was in a bit of a hurry I couldn't wait for the next car, so I punched in my floor and tried not to breathe deeply. The elevator went up one floor, stopped, and the four people got off. I had two more floors to go. When I got there, and the doors opened, there were three people waiting to get in. There I was in the elevator by myself in all that stink. I couldn't look them in the eyes as I got off. In my mind, I was screaming, *It wasn't me. I'm innocent!* I can only imagine what those folks had to say about our anesthesia department, and me, to everybody they knew.

All the ladies in ICU laughed like crazy when I told them what had happened. So did the whole OR when I got back.

The good news: The patient I intubated in ICU did fine.

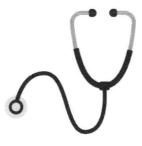

17. Brushing Teeth

In 2002 I worked at a large hospital in St. Petersburg, Florida, with a mixed group of CRNAs and anesthesiologists. One early afternoon I was notified of an add-on case in my schedule: a thirty-five-year-old woman with Ludwig's angina. This is an infection that starts inside the mouth and spreads rapidly through the adjacent connective and soft tissues to the jaw and even down into the neck forming large abscesses. A frequent cause is poor oral hygiene. The oral surgeon doing the surgery and draining the abscesses told me that the lady hadn't brushed her teeth for many years, which had caused the infection.

When I arrived in preop, I saw that our patient had a large swelling on the right side of her face, extending down toward the jaw. She was obviously in some discomfort but very friendly. The first question I asked after looking over her chart and introducing myself was why she hadn't brushed her teeth for years. "Because it hurt so much when I did it that I quit" was her reply. I assured her that we would take good care of her but that she might wake up with a breathing tube in place. She needn't worry, though, because it was just a precaution and we'd take it out as soon as we could. The rest of her health history was unremarkable.

Airway management is always the primary focus of any form of anesthesia, but when the surgery is in and around the patient's airway it's critical. I had her open her mouth as wide as she could to ascertain whether there was enough room to get a breathing tube through it and into her windpipe. Based on my inspection, the opening appeared to be adequate.

We brought the lady to the OR and after she was anesthetized, I had no trouble getting my breathing tube in place. The inside of her mouth was inflamed and puffy, with areas of pus around her lower right molars. The oral surgeon said he hadn't seen a case this bad in years and that this lady was in for a long period of treatment. He worked inside her mouth and outside along her jaw, draining and irrigating out all the pus for the better part of an hour. We also had antibiotics running in her IV. At the end of the case her facial swelling was considerably decreased, and I was able to take the breathing tube out and wake her up. In the recovery room, she did fine.

Two days later, the first scheduled case in my room was the same lady. This time, we were to perform a debridement (removal of dead tissue) of the neck and upper chest. The infection that had started in her mouth now extended into the soft tissues of her neck and upper chest and was gradually destroying them. This time, when I saw her she was in a preop isolation room and was frightened, crying, and hot from fever. Her neck and chest were covered with heavy dressings because of copious amounts of purulent drainage.

I gave her some light sedation, and we got her back to the OR quickly. The same oral surgeon was assigned to the case, along with a plastic surgeon to assist in case she needed skin grafting. Again, her airway was adequate, and after anesthetizing her I was able to get a breathing tube in without any problem. When the dressings came off it was a horrible sight. Her neck and upper chest down to her nipples was all dark-purple and black, with tissue sloughing off and exuding heavy, foul drainage. In many places dead tissue could be seen down to her chest wall.

The two surgeons worked for over an hour, removing all that tissue and irrigating it away. After they had finished, her chest from chin to nipples and all the way to both shoulders was completely denuded and raw. No consideration was given to doing any skin grafts at that point because the area involved was too large and probably still full of bacteria. Due to the extensive nature of her surgery and how sick she was, I decided to leave her breathing tube in place and bring her to the recovery room to be put on the ventilator. She stayed there for an hour and was later discharged to an isolation room in ICU. I checked on her later in the day. Because she had been having some hypotension issues, probably due to sepsis, there was a potent IV blood pressure medication running in a pump to correct it. She still had the breathing tube in place and was on the ventilator and sedated.

The next morning, after getting ready for my cases, I went to ICU to check on her again. She had died during the night! That really shocked me and I had to go collect myself for a bit.

All from not brushing her teeth...

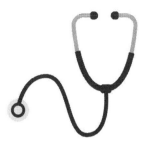

18. Train Tracks

In 1976 I got called to the hospital by the supervisor on a cold, fall Saturday night in Bemidji, for a traumatic amputation. When I got there the ambulance was just arriving from with a sixteen-year-old Native American boy in a state of unconscious shock from massive hemorrhage. It was a horrible sight. His complexion was grayish, he was covered with blood and had multiple traumatic amputations and facial lacerations. His right arm had been severed above the elbow, his left arm was missing just below the elbow, and both legs were gone just below the knees—the OR term for that is spaghetti arms and legs. He also had multiple deep facial lacerations.

I felt his neck and found a weak carotid pulse. As we were getting him into the ER the ambulance driver told us that he'd been found on the railroad tracks and looked like he had been in a drunken stupor and placed there by someone. I quickly got a breathing tube into his windpipe, started large-bore IVs on each side of his neck in the external jugular veins, and drew blood for a type and crossmatch and lab work. The surgeon put tourniquets around his stumps, and I ran to the operating room to get set up, telling the supervisor to call Minneapolis and have them send their plane up to get him in the morning. When we got him to the OR I could only get a pediatric blood pressure cuff way up high on what was left of his left arm and a precordial stethoscope taped to his chest right over his heart. The stethoscope attached to an earpiece placed in my ear so I could monitor his heartbeat continually.

I couldn't get a readable blood pressure but could always hear an ongoing heartbeat and feel an extremely weak carotid pulse. After two liters of rapidly infused warm normal saline, I finally got a blood pressure reading of about

40 over 20. The surgeon was working fast, cleaning up his stumps, stopping the bleeding, and cutting away damaged tissue on his extremities, while the circulating nurse gingerly cleaned up the lacerations on his face. He had one huge laceration all across his forehead just above the eyebrows that had turned a flap loose and partially flipped up over the top of his head. Fortunately, his eyes were still intact, but one cheek had a deep gash in it. The other had a large flap loose that hung down over his jawbone. His lips were all cut up, and he had no intact upper or lower teeth—just a few broken-off snags. His nose was squashed but still attached to his face, and one ear was ripped about halfway off of his head.

When the lab work came back, his hemoglobin was extremely low from blood loss at the scene and in the ambulance, meanwhile I pumped three units of warm whole blood into him. Finally, his blood pressure came up to a low normal and he started making urine through his catheter. For the next six hours we worked on sewing up his facial lacerations and repairing his extremity stumps. I was able to pass a stomach tube through his mouth and, fortunately, there wasn't much down there except liquid.

When we finished, the kid looked much better. His vital signs were stable, his skin color was good, and we able to take him to ICU for emergence from anesthesia. I decided to leave the breathing tube in and although he was breathing on his own, he wasn't awake and I didn't want to have any airway issues when he finally did wake up. All the alcohol in his system combined with the anesthetics would take a while to wear off. I stayed with him in ICU all night.

Finally, early in the morning, he started to wake up a little, and I was able to remove his breathing tube and let him breathe oxygen through a mask. He was very disoriented and in a lot of pain, so I sedated him with narcotics and he drifted in and out of consciousness. About mid-morning the air ambulance from Minneapolis arrived and the nurse who came with it was amazed at what had happened and all we'd done. When the rescue team took him we all breathed a sigh of relief that he was going to be okay.

About nine months later, while my wife and I were shopping at the little mall in town, I noticed a person in a wheelchair by the food court coming toward me. I could hardly believe who it was: our sixteen-year-old patient with the spaghetti arms and legs whom we'd sent to Minneapolis almost a year before. He had prosthetic legs and arms now and his face showed the results of what had obviously been an excellent job of plastic surgery. He looked happy, even smiling and laughing as he was being wheeled around. I didn't speak to him because I was sure he wouldn't know me plus the memories of that fateful night might not be something he'd have cared to revisit. I was so glad that he was all fixed up, back home, and apparently adjusted to his situation. They had done a good job on him in Minneapolis. It was rewarding to see that all our efforts that night had paid off.

Two weeks later, he was found with a bullet hole between his eyes.

Somebody had wanted him dead.

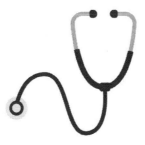

19. "I Resent That"

In 2003 I was called to a hospital Cardiac ICU one afternoon to start an arterial line on a patient. This procedure is done by inserting a catheter into the radial artery on the bottom of the patient's wrist and hooking it up to a pressurized and transduced saline line for measuring their vital signs, pulse and blood pressure with every heartbeat. It's a useful monitoring tool for critically ill patients.

When I arrived at the room I found an agitated, confused, hallucinating and vocal, elderly lady garbling continually, with several IVs running and in four-point leather restraints lying in bed. She was obviously in DTs (delirium tremens—alcohol withdrawal symptoms). The nurse attending her said that she had been a nursing supervisor at the hospital years ago.

Her present state was quite a sight and as we stood next to her bed I asked the nurse, "What have we got going here, a Korsakoff's?" This is a syndrome most frequently caused by the neurotoxic effects of chronic alcoholism. The nurse said that was exactly what it was. In the one lucid moment the lady probably experienced in all her current hallucinatory confusion, she turned to me and yelled out, "I resent that, you f*cking asshole!" Then she slipped right back into oblivion. That gave both of us a huge laugh. I started the arterial line and left. For a long time afterward, whenever that nurse and I saw each other, our greeting was, "How're you doing, FA?"

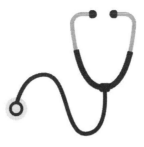

20. The Chick Table

To fix a broken hip, many orthopedic surgeons use a special operating room fracture table called a Chick table and at first glance, this table might seem like something out of the Spanish Inquisition. It's designed with a platform for resting the patient's upper body on, with a small platform for the buttocks and a stirrup for each foot on a screw mount, which the feet are securely fastened into. When a hip is fractured, generally there is a shortening of the leg on the affected side. To be able to return the leg and hip to its normal anatomical position for repair, the leg has traction applied to it which stretches it into position so the surgeon is able to insert a titanium pin into it, fixing it permanently.

To obtain the required traction, a perineal post is fastened to the lower end of the buttock platform, which sticks up between the patient's legs in their crotch so that when the stirrup on the affected leg is screwed out, it lengthens the leg by pulling it against the perineal post. Needless to say, the patient's perineum is well padded for this procedure. Also, a heavy nylon strap is placed across the patient's chest to secure their upper body on the table. In essence, the only things holding the patient on the table are the foot stirrups, the perineal post on the buttock platform, and the chest strap. The patient is always well anesthetized before any of this type of positioning is done.

On a late afternoon, we had an elderly, extremely confused, and debilitated lady with a fractured left hip as an add on case. Except for advanced dementia, her health history was stable enough that we felt confident about successfully performing her surgery. I put her to sleep on the gurney and then we carefully transferred her to the Chick table and got her positioned, prepped, and draped.

We elevated the table about four feet to accommodate our six-foot, four-inch surgeon.

The surgery went well and only took about an hour. After it was finished, the patient was waking up on the Chick table, and as we were taking the surgical drapes off she mumbled something to the circulating nurse.

The nurse said to me, "She says the strap across her chest is too tight."

I replied, "Don't take that strap off because the perineal post has been removed, and that's the only thing holding her on the table!"

I turned to get something off my anesthesia cart, and as I did I heard a thunk—the kind of sound you might hear if you dropped a cantaloupe or small watermelon on your kitchen floor. I spun around and horror of horrors, the circulator had taken the chest strap off and our poor old lady had fallen off the table and hit her head on the marble floor from four feet in the air. To make matters worse, her feet were still fastened into the stirrups, so she was dangling by her feet at a forty-five degree angle with her head and shoulders on the floor.

I yelled at the nurse, "What in the hell did you just do?" The nurse just stood there with a blank stare. I said, "Get the hell out in the hall and get us some help and get our surgeon in here immediately."

The scrub technician for the case was from Poland and new in America. He didn't have a good command of English, but he knew enough to quickly scoop our patient off the floor and hoist her back up on the table. I told him to strap her down, hold onto her, and not to let the circulator anywhere near her. The lady was awake now and screaming gibberish, so I had to give her a small dose of sedation. I couldn't understand the Polish our scrub tech was saying, but it looked like he was praying.

The surgeon came into the room, exclaiming, "Oh, my god. Oh, my god. What the hell happened here? Get X-Ray up here immediately."

Now the room was a flurry of activity. When the x-ray technician arrived with a C-arm fluoroscope, we x-rayed our patient from one end to the other for the better part of an hour. As luck would have it, we couldn't find a thing wrong with her. The surgeon was still mad but said that we were very lucky and that this may have been a case of Divine intervention, since if she were ever able to tell anybody what had happened nobody would likely believe her because she was so confused.

That was the circulating nurse's last day in the operating room.

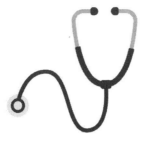

21. Esophageal Varicies

Chronic long-term alcoholism causes many health problems, not the least of which is cirrhosis of the liver. In advanced cases of cirrhosis, the liver becomes full of scar tissue and its many functions are then impaired, causing blood circulation through it to be impeded and leading to esophageal varicies—varicose veins in the esophagus. These veins are very fragile and can rupture easily and spontaneously. When this happens, it's an emergency situation, since massive bleeding usually occurs out of the person's mouth and, if left unchecked, the patient will bleed to death. One treatment for esophageal variceal rupture in the '70s was to insert a large multi-lumen balloon catheter called the Sengstaken-Blakemore tube into the patient's esophagus. When inflated the balloon puts pressure against the ruptured area(s) to stop the bleeding.

Our little hospital had its own blood bank which kept a selection of all the blood types on hand. Some blood types are more uncommon than others, and the blood bank usually just had one unit of those available because they outdated frequently and would call in donors if they needed more. It happened that our town drunk had one of those uncommon blood types, which was the same as mine (A negative) and a few other folks in town. He was a pleasant fellow, but every year it seemed, in the dead of our northern Minnesota winters, he'd show up in the emergency room bleeding profusely from his esophageal varicies. Also, every year, we'd have to call all the donors in with his blood type to donate for him. It wasn't uncommon to have to give him four or five units of whole blood by the time his bleeding was under control.

was always a mess in the emergency room, covered with blood coming of both ends. We had to work fast getting him to the OR so we could get Blakemore tube in him and get it stopped. As you might expect, maintaining his airway under these circumstances was crucial. Each time, I had my circulating nurse suck the blood out of his mouth so I could see to get a breathing tube in his trachea to seal off his airway. He was usually in shock and so weak and barely conscious that he couldn't put up much resistance.

Once the Blakemore tube was in place and inflated and the bleeding controlled, we could empty his stomach. I kept a large-bore IV running to give him fluid to hold his blood pressure up, and when the blood was ready we would transfuse him until he was stable. It's absolutely amazing what the effect of a few units of freshly drawn, warm whole blood has on a person in his condition. Within the hour he was pretty much wide awake, responding to commands, and aware of his circumstance. After a while we could very carefully remove the Blakemore tube, and almost always the bleeding had stopped by then. He would spend the night in ICU and a few days on the ward afterward.

There is always a chance that a chronic alcoholic might go into DTs from alcohol withdrawal, which has a significant mortality rate, and to keep that from happening back in those days, the doctor would order a 5 percent solution of alcohol to be run in his IV, which kept him pretty happy.

This sequence of events went on for five years. Whether I was on call or not, I was always called in to donate a unit of blood for him and it always seemed to be on a cold winter night. One year, when they called me to donate, I was so sick with the flu that I couldn't make it. He died during that episode. I doubt that not getting a unit of my blood was the reason, I think his body just couldn't take any more insult.

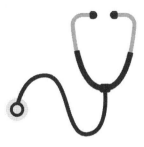

22. Farm Accident

We were notified one cold winter's afternoon in February that a farm accident victim with a bad leg injury was coming in from a small town twenty-five miles west of Bemidji. When the ambulance arrived, they had a barely conscious young boy with his right leg wrapped in many layers of bloody dressings from groin to ankle. The ambulance driver told us that he had been driving a tractor out in the field, spreading manure from the cow barn, when a large chunk of frozen manure got stuck in the tines of the spreader and locked it up. He stopped the tractor and went back to free up the tines but had neglected to disengage the power takeoff. He kicked the manure chunk to get it loose, and when it popped free, the large tines started spinning and caught his boot, pulling his whole leg into them before they locked up again. Somehow he managed to free himself, get back on the tractor, and drive himself off the field. What a monumental effort that must have been.

We quickly got him into the emergency room, and I started two large-bore IVs for lab work and warmed normal saline fluids while the nurses cut off his snowmobile suit and clothes. His right leg from groin to foot was a real mess. Thankfully, his genitals were unharmed. All the soft tissue left in the injured area was severely lacerated and bleeding, with manure, his clothing, and remnants of boot ground into it. Luckily, his femoral artery was intact, though totally denuded and faintly pulsating. If that had been severed the young kid probably would have died out in the field. We wrapped him in warm blankets and quickly took him to the OR. By the time I got him anesthetized the blood and lab work were ready. He was anemic, having probably lost close to three units of blood on the tractor and in the spreader.

We worked on him for three hours, cutting away dead tissue, irrigating debris and manure out of his wounds, and controlling the bleeding. I transfused him with three units of warm whole blood, so that by the end of the case he was stable and had good vital signs. His leg was quite a sight. There wasn't more than a few inches of normal skin anywhere, and a lot of muscle had been destroyed. He woke up in a lot of pain and in the recovery room we gave him narcotics and antibiotics. Amazingly, he could still wiggle his toes.

The surgeon called Minneapolis to send their air ambulance.

I didn't hear anything more about that case until six months later, when the doctor from that little town called us to say he was home and doing well. He walked with a slight limp but, miracles of miracles, had no infections during the whole course of his treatment.

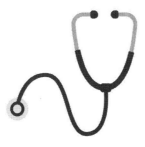

23. The Mixer

I received a call from the emergency room one afternoon in the late '70s. A patient there had a most unusual injury and would probably be coming to surgery they said. As I entered the ER, I could hear a great deal of moaning coming from one of the stalls. Our patient was an elderly gentleman with an apparatus in his lap that looked like a large industrial mixer—the kind on your kitchen countertop that mixes everything in the bowl all by itself. Turns out that Grandpa was sitting in a living room easy chair with the mixer in his lap, trying to see what was wrong with it. He and his wife were babysitting their three-year-old granddaughter that day.

The mixer cord was hanging over the edge of the chair while he was tinkering with it and, unbeknownst to him, his little granddaughter walked by, saw the cord and plugged it into a wall outlet right next to the chair. The mixer immediately started up with a fury in Grandpa's lap and the beaters grabbed his pants in the crotch area, grinding them and everything underneath—namely his genitals—into their tines until they locked up tight. Poor Grandpa was helpless and in agony! His wife called an ambulance immediately.

We brought him to the OR, where I anesthetized him on the ER cart. After he was asleep, the surgeon was able to disconnect the mixer shafts from the motor, but the tines of the beater blades were locked so tightly in his pants that we had to call the head of maintenance to come up with a bolt cutter and take the blades apart piecemeal. It was quite a sight: heavy-duty side cutters and surgical scissors working side by side with all the operators being very careful not to injure whatever anatomy was involved underneath.

Finally, Grandpa's crotch was disengaged from the mixer and the surgeon gingerly removed the last little pieces of his pants and underwear. Amazingly, his genitals appeared to be unharmed but were lacerated, very swollen, and discolored. The surgeon palpated everything and was satisfied that his anatomy, pending x-ray, was intact so he proceeded to clean everything and sew up all the small lacerations. We put antibiotics in his IV and applied an ice pack to the area when we were done.

Epilogue:

Grandpa's genitalia x-rays were all negative, and after a night in the hospital he went home with an ice bag and lots of pain medication and Grandma went out to buy a new mixer.

Many years later, I saw Grandpa downtown. He said everything was fine and that whenever they had a family gathering and that story came up, his granddaughter—now in her twenties—would turn beet-red with embarrassment and leave the room…which would make everybody laugh even harder.

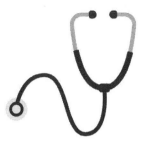

24. Popeye

I had an unexpected surprise one morning while finishing up a routine laparoscopic gall bladder case on a healthy middle-aged man. I had spoken with him in preop, and he had assured me that he'd had no problems with any of his previous surgeries or general anesthetics. He had normal airway anatomy, was not on any medications, and had no chronic health conditions.

For laparoscopic surgery the patient needs to have a breathing tube (endotracheal tube) placed into their windpipe, which seals it off after they're anesthetized, so that no stomach contents can get into their airway. It also enables them to be adequately ventilated if they're placed in an awkward position. Sterile ophthalmic ointment is placed in the patient's eyes, which are then sealed shut with non-allergenic tape to make sure they're protected underneath the drapes.

The case took about forty-five minutes and was uneventful. As the dressings were being applied, and I was waking the man up, I gently removed his eye tapes and the endotracheal tube. As the tube slid passed his vocal cords he gave a moderate cough, whereupon his right eye popped right out of its socket! It flopped down on his lower eyelid, hanging by the cords attached to it. I let out a yelp and jumped back. The surgeon had left the room, but the rest of the OR staff came running over and were aghast!

Immediately, I called for some sterile saline and gloves and irrigated the fellow's eye socket while gently placing the eyeball back into it. I taped the lid shut, put sterile gauze over it, and called for the surgeon and my attending anesthesiologist. They both came in, took a look, and determined that he'd have to see an ophthalmologist before he left the hospital. I brought the fellow to the recovery room and explained what had happened to his nurse and about that time he woke up.

I told him what had happened and that his eyelid was taped shut and not to remove the tape. His comment was priceless: "Yeah, that happens a lot when I cough or sneeze, so whenever I feel one coming on I have to hold my hand over my eye to keep that from happening. I can even make it happen if I hold my breath and bear down." I told him that I wished he'd said that preop because it gave me and the OR staff quite a scare and my attending anesthesiologist wanted him to see an ophthalmologist now. He just laughed and told me not to worry about it.

Back in 1952 I managed to get into a freak show at the Minnesota State Fair. They had a guy there called Popeye who came out on stage and made both of his eyes pop out of their sockets the same way my patient's eye had. Popeye walked around like that and then just reached up and stuck them back in while people in the crowd gasped and shrieked. I could even hear a few retching.

Just when you think you've seen it all...

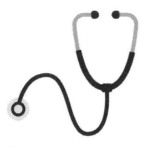

25. Coffee in the Locker Room

Early one morning I was sitting on the couch in the locker room of our little hospital's surgery department all by myself with a cup of coffee and waiting for my first case of the day to arrive in the preop department. The room was pretty small, and I was leaning way back with my feet up high resting on the lockers in front of me. I was sipping coffee and daydreaming when suddenly I got a big gulp of coffee in my airway. My reflex action was to take a deep breath which, of course, drew it right onto my vocal cords and caused a massive laryngospasm—an uncontrolled involuntary muscular contraction of the vocal cords—causing partial or complete obstruction of the airway. This is usually caused by some foreign substance; i.e., swallowing the wrong way.

As I struggled to get a breath, knowing full well what was happening, my mind raced with the overriding thought that I'd lived my whole life up until now only to die in an obscure locker room all alone. I was scared and flailing a little, trying to cough to clear my airway and be able to breathe. Of course, I couldn't make a sound for somebody to hear me. I tried to stand up, and in the process fell over sideways on the couch which turned out to be a stroke of luck. My fall caused the coffee to run out of my airway and mouth and allowed me the tiniest breath. I let out a small cough, which cleared the rest of my airway. I gasped in a great, big breath, followed by a fit of coughing. There was a knock at the door and a voice asked, "Are you all right?" I gasped, "Yes, now I am. Just swallowed wrong."

In all my years in anesthesia, I've seen and treated many laryngospasms that have occurred for different reasons, but every one of those patients were in the OR and either completely or partially anesthetized and had no conscious awareness of it. Outside of the OR, I once saw a surgeon friend perform the Heimlich maneuver to clear an airway on a fellow in the cafeteria who was purple and struggling with food caught in his throat. Once, I did mouth-to-mouth resuscitation on a friend who'd had a heart attack during a party, but that was my only personal experience with such an issue.

Looking back, I think if anything besides coffee had obstructed my airway, the staff may have ultimately found me in the locker room dead on the couch.

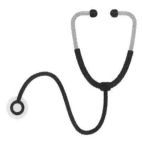

26. Knock Me Out

My first case of the day one morning in the late '80s was a relatively minor gynecologic procedure on a young gal. She was with her husband in preop and they both had a good sense of humor so we laughed and joked a bit. It was the first time she'd ever had general anesthesia, and the one (not uncommon) concern she had was that she wouldn't be asleep when they started or that she might wake up before the procedure was over. I assured her that I would not let that happen under any circumstance and not to worry about it.

When the time came to bring her to the OR, I gave her a small dose of tranquilizer in her IV. After she was anesthetized, I administered a dose of a short-acting narcotic which I thought, along with the tranquilizer she'd had in preop, would allow her to wake up after the procedure and be lightly sedated and fairly comfortable. The procedure went well and was over in a half hour. She was barely awake as we moved her from the OR table to the gurney but would take a deep breath when I asked her to. We were in the OR located at the end of a hall and farthest away from the recovery room.

As the circulating nurse and I started down the hall with her, she woke up quite a bit more, gave her surroundings a disoriented look, and started screaming at the top of her lungs, *"Knock me the f*ck out! Knock me the f*ck out!"* I told her repeatedly that she was just waking up, but it didn't seem to register at all. You can imagine the reactions of the people in the hallway as we went by. Some were laughing; others gave us horrified looks. People in other operating rooms were looking out their doors aghast. I hadn't brought any medication with me to sedate her, so we hustled down the hall. When we arrived at the recovery room, and the automatic doors swung open, she was still screaming those same words which snapped all the nurses—along with a few wide-awake patients—to attention.

I shouted to quickly get me some Versed, the mild tranquilizer I'd given her in preop, so I could calm her down until she was fully awake. Unfortunately, there wasn't an isolation room to put her in so she had to remain there, screaming, oblivious to whatever was said to her until I had titrated enough Versed into the IV to let her drift off in a pleasant slumber. While all this was going on the recovery room nurses moved all the conscious patients out into the hallway. My patient dozed for another hour and finally woke up with no recollection of what had happened.

I've had many patients over the years wake up after their operation and wonder when they're going to go to sleep, but I never had another patient like her. I still think about it and laugh.

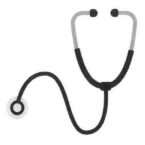

27. Two Carotid Stories

Every person has a carotid artery on each side of their neck that supplies blood to the brain and head. When these arteries become severely narrowed because of plaque buildup, the chances of stroke are greatly increased. Quite often the recommended treatment is carotid endarterectomy, a procedure during which a surgeon clamps the affected carotid below the narrowing, opens it up and removes the plaque that's causing the blockage and then closes it securely and unclamps it. Modern carotid endarterectomy surgical technique also involves the use of an electroencephalogram (EEG) while the vessel is clamped to monitor a patient's brain activity during the surgery. If it shows the least bit of brain compromise, the surgeon immediately inserts a shunt around the clamp to establish adequate blood flow to the brain. This process wasn't always used. As recently as fifteen years ago, not all surgeons used the EEG when performing this kind of surgery.

Anesthetic requirements for carotid surgery are intense. The patient has an arterial catheter placed in one of the radial arteries of either wrist to measure their blood pressure and pulse. It is connected to a pulse and pulse wave transducer and with each heartbeat it gives a digital readout on the anesthesia monitor screen. There is also an EKG monitor, an oxygen saturation monitor, and an esophageal probe for temperature monitoring. The arms are tucked by the patient's sides so the surgeon and his assistant have easy access to the patient's neck. Along with keeping the patient asleep, the main focus of an anesthesia provider is to keep the patient's blood pressure within that patient's normal range to slightly on the high side of that. Considering that one of their carotids will be clamped, decreasing the blood flow that it may have provided to the brain otherwise, high or low blood pressure at any time during the procedure could precipitate a brain injury. Thus, we keep an armamentarium of drugs in our anesthesia carts to correct any of those situations, should they develop.

Late one afternoon I was administering anesthesia to an elderly man for carotid surgery. The surgeon was a very experienced fellow who had been in practice for a long time, had done many of these procedures, and was not using the EEG. The surgery was proceeding well, the carotid was exposed, and all the patient's vital signs were stable. The surgeon called for a carotid clamp, alerted everyone to get ready, and clamped it. Just after the clamp was applied, the surgeon's cell phone, which was sitting over on a side table, rang. Without looking up he asked the circulating nurse who was calling. She looked at the phone and told him it was his wife. With that, he said, "I'll take it," broke scrub, walked over to the table, picked up the phone and headed for the door to the hall. As he walked by me, I heard him say, "Tell them to come over to our house, and we can all ride together."

Now, mind you, the patient's carotid is clamped and the clamp is straight up in the air moving back and forth like a metronome with every heartbeat while the surgeon is out in the hall. We all stared at each other, amazed that he had the nerve to leave a patient in that circumstance. I watched the clock. He was gone for a full nine minutes which seemed like an eternity to us. When he came back, he was jovial as if nothing had happened. He finished the surgery. The patient woke up fine, was oriented to time and place and could move all his extremities. Disaster averted!

My first case of the day a few years ago was a carotid endarterectomy on an obese elderly man with a significantly occluded right carotid artery and who also had a history of hypertension and diabetes. It was to be performed by the most talented surgeon I've ever had the pleasure of working with in my whole career. He used the EEG monitor and had performed many of these operations from incision to dressings in less than one hour. The rest of our surgical team that day were all very experienced OR personnel and had done many such cases. The circulating nurse was a retired Army male nurse who was quite experienced and who took every opportunity to let us know that.

The case was progressing well, but the patient's blood pressure tended to be somewhat labile—a little high one minute and a little low the next. I was able to control it by adjusting my anesthetic gas concentration. As mentioned, for this type of surgery the patient's arms are tucked by their sides so the surgeon and his assistant have easy access to the neck. Just before clamping the carotid artery the patient needs an intravenous dose of heparin (an anticoagulant) to keep their blood from clotting as protection against brain injury. When the surgeon was ready to clamp the carotid, he gave me the go-ahead for heparin, and I injected a dose into his IV.

The carotid was clamped, and right away the patient's blood pressure became even more unstable than it had been. I administered medication in the form of an intravenous bolus and infusion to correct it, with only marginal success. I also increased and decreased the concentration of my inhalation anesthetic gas as an adjunct to the IV medication. I was just barely keeping the patient's blood pressure within the limits of acceptability at that point and was perplexed as to why the meds I was giving didn't seem to be working well. This scenario lasted for about another fifteen minutes, until the surgeon had finished removing the plaque, closed the carotid, and was ready to unclamp it. Once that happened, my patient's blood pressure settled down and was much easier to control, so I was able to discontinue the medication infusion.

About that time, the circulating nurse, who was standing by the side of the OR table, said, "Ron, look at this puddle of fluid on the floor by where his arm is tucked. I bet his IV is leaking."

I immediately hollered out, "Get that arm untucked right now and have a look!"

The surgical team moved out of the way so the nurse could get the patient's arm on an arm board. Sure enough, the IV tubing had become disconnected from the catheter in his vein and IV fluid had been running into the drapes and on the floor during the entire case. That explained why my blood pressure meds hadn't been working but, worse yet, the patient had not received that heparin anticoagulant I'd administered just prior to the carotid being clamped. With a great deal of trepidation I told my surgeon friend what had happened, and he said, "I thought something was funny, the way the carotid snapped back after I unclamped it."

That was a stressful time, because all the scenarios of this patient waking up with a compromised brain from a blood clot raced through my mind and it took another long ten minutes for the case to finish so I could wake him up. As our patient came out of the anesthetic, I called his name. He opened his eyes. I told him to lift up his head and take a deep breath and he did so. The surgeon had him squeeze both of his hands and wiggle his feet. The patient did both successfully. He also told us his name, age, date, and his wife's name. I announced to the staff with a huge sigh of relief that we'd dodged a bullet and our patient was okay! The only comment the surgeon made, in his distinctive Irish brogue, was "All's well that ends well, Ron!"

After I came back from the recovery room, I was angry as hell with the circulator. I asked him why a so-called experienced OR nurse, as he had claimed to be, didn't say something about that large puddle on the floor as it was forming underneath the patient's tucked arm during the case. I told him that it was right there in front of where he was sitting on his stool and had obviously been accumulating for a while (expletives deleted). His response was a blank stare. Then he walked away.

He quit about a month later. Good riddance!

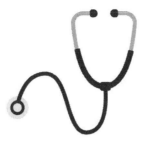

28. Worried I Won't Wake Up

Everyone's nervous when they're about to undergo surgery. Some people, however, are nervous to a fault and can barely hold it together, even in preop. Such was the case with a middle-aged lady patient of mine one morning. After looking over her chart, I approached the cubicle and noticed that she was with her husband and looked frightened. I introduced myself and asked her how she was.

"I'm so worried and scared," she replied. I asked her why she was so upset and she said, "I'm afraid of the anesthesia and that I won't ever wake up from it." I had to think for a minute. I didn't want to use any of the old standard lines about that never happening, because nobody believes it anyway, so I said, "Are you in luck today!" Now I had their full attention. "We just had an anesthesia department meeting this morning, and the chief announced a new policy going into effect immediately. We can't charge you unless you wake up, so now we have an incentive."

You should have seen their faces. The lady was clearly shocked and surprised and her husband broke out in a huge belly laugh. After a minute she started to giggle too and calmed down. That was all it took, and with a little tranquilizer in her IV she was very comfortable as we went to the OR.

I thought later about what might've happened if I had misjudged that couple. My remarks could've had the opposite effect and caused big trouble for me, the department, and the hospital.

She woke up perfectly after her surgery.

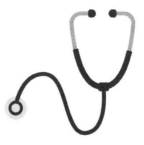

29. The Thermostat

Back in the 1970s, just after I became a CRNA, I worked at a large private hospital in a suburb of Minneapolis. It had a big OR with ten surgical suites and a dental suite located quite a distance away from the main OR. The chief of all anesthesia services then was an irascible old anesthesiologist who'd been there a long time and fought many political battles with hospital administrators and medical staffs over the years but he ran an excellent department and had an accomplished chief CRNA in charge of it. The dental room was used predominately for pediatric cases on children who needed a lot of work.

I was assigned to the dental room one morning for two cases with a very friendly pediatric dentist. Our first patient was a cute little seven-year-old boy who was very cooperative and "blew up the balloon" to drift off to sleep. After he was anesthetized I started his IV, put an endotracheal tube in his trachea and the case got underway. The room temperature was a little cool, so the dentist asked our circulator to please turn up the heat a bit. After about an hour my attending anesthesiologist, who was the big chief, showed up to see how everything was going. The very first thing he said when he walked in was "Who in the hell turned the heat up in this room?" The dentist told him that he thought it was a little bit too cold in there, so he had the circulator do it. The chief said, "Nobody touches this thermostat and moves it from where I have it set."

With that he walked over and turned the thermostat down to where it had been and left. The dentist said to the circulator, "Go look out in the hall and see if he's gone." She did so and came back, reporting that he had indeed gone back to the OR, whereupon the dentist told her to turn the thermostat back up to where he wanted it. I knew exactly what was going to happen, and it was only a matter of time before the confrontation.

A half hour later, the chief showed up again, walked over to the thermostat, turned it down, and said to the dentist, "Keep your damn hands off this thermostat." He left the room, and the dentist told the circulator to please turn the thermostat up again, but she refused, saying that she was afraid to and didn't want to get in the middle of things—and besides, she had to see the chief every day while the dentist only came there occasionally.

The dentist stood up to go turn the thermostat up himself at about the same time the chief came back into the room-carrying a toolbox and cordless drill with him. Without saying a word, he walked over to the thermostat, put a bit in the drill, and drilled a hole through the thermostat adjustment lever and into the wall. Next, he pulled out a long screw, put it through the adjustment lever and into the wall. He turned to the dentist with a vehement look and left. Nobody said much for a few minutes. Finally, the dentist announced, "After my next case, I won't be back here ever again."

Throughout my career, the temperature in the OR has always been a bone of contention, although these days the surgeon has the final say. Studies have shown that patients do not do well if they get cold during a procedure, and the Joint Commission on Hospital Accreditation has criteria for determining optimal surgical patient temperature levels. We have many ways to keep patients warm now, from continuous warm airflow blanket coverings to heated IV fluids. Also, basic standard of care now dictates that all anesthesia providers monitor the temperatures of their anesthetized patients. Cold rooms these days are only a problem for the OR staff, and on long cases it's not unusual to see a few of them wrapped in blankets from the department's warming cabinet.

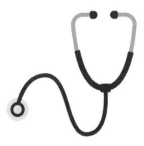

30. The Wrong Room

Forty-five years ago in our little northern Minnesota hospital, we had an ophthalmologist working there who performed cataract surgery. He used general anesthesia for all his cases, unlike the modern-day techniques of local anesthesia plus sedation. Most of his patients were elderly and his surgeries always took a minimum of two hours per case. All surgical patients were admitted to the hospital the night before to undergo whatever preparations they might need, and our policy then was whichever CRNA was on call would go in to make preop rounds on them.

One evening while making my rounds, I decided to start with the cataract patients. I gathered up their charts, looked them over, and proceeded to each patient's room for a discussion of their anesthesia. The first patient I saw was an elderly lady lying quietly in bed watching TV with her roommate. I called her name and she mumbled something. I introduced myself, announcing that I was from the anesthesia department and would be putting her to sleep for her cataract operation the next day so that the doctor could fix her eye and she'd be able to see again. I was not prepared for her response. She sat straight up in bed and started shouting, "I'll be able to see again? Oh, thank you, Jesus! Thank you, God! I'll be able to see again! Thank you! Thank you! Thank you! My prayers have been answered! Thank you, Jesus. I'll be able to see again. I'll see again!"

This really surprised me, since this ophthalmologist's patients were always well informed about their surgery beforehand—I was never the first one to tell them about it. The lady went on loudly thanking God and Jesus and I couldn't get in a word of explanation to her. Finally, I left the room and went to the nurses' station to ask the charge nurse what on earth was going on. I explained that after I told the lady about her cataract surgery and vision improvement, she went crazy. The nurse gasped and said, "Oh, my god. You didn't just say it to that woman, did you? That's not the right patient. She's confused and in for diabetic retinopathy."

I replied, "Yes, I did. How on earth could that have happened?"

I showed her the surgery schedule and the patient's chart, which had corresponding names and room numbers. The minute she saw it, she gasped again and said, "They changed her room on the last shift and obviously didn't change her chart around. Did you look at her name band?"

That hit me like an electric shock. I hadn't! I had broken the cardinal rule of patient identification. By not properly checking everything, I wound up accidentally speaking to a lady who was in no condition to hear what I had just told her. I really felt terrible and was embarrassed since now the nurse had to call her doctor, whom I knew quite well, and explain the situation in order to get some sedation for the poor woman.

The next morning, before surgery, I checked with the night shift, who told me that the lady had been awake every hour thanking Jesus that her vision was going to be fixed in the morning. When I saw her doctor I apologized profusely.

And I never made that mistake again.

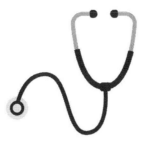

31. The Snowplow

From 1971 to 1987 I lived in northern Minnesota, ninety miles south of Ontario, on twenty acres of thick woods located twelve miles from town. The house was set back from the main road about two blocks at the end of a long, winding, dirt driveway. It was a gorgeous pastoral setting but the winters could be inclement with temperatures often thirty below zero and lots of deep snow. Fortunately, I had a friend from town who would plow my driveway every time it snowed so I could get to the hospital when I was on call.

On a bitter cold Friday evening in the early 1970s, while I was on call, a raging blizzard came down unleashing enough snowfall and wind to plug up the end of my driveway and make it impassable. During this blizzard, at about 9 p.m., I got a call from the hospital needing me to come in for an emergency appendectomy. My friend from town hadn't been out to plow yet, cell phones weren't on the market and I didn't have a snowmobile. I was in a quandary. I decided to call the sheriff to see if they could help. The friendly dispatcher who answered told me she'd see what she could do and call me right back. About fifteen minutes later she called back. "Mr. Whitchurch," she said, "if you can bundle up and make it to the end of your driveway, we're going to send one of the county plows for you. If that's okay, they'll be out there in about fifteen minutes." I said, "You betcha," and hustled to get into my winter parka and boots.

It was tough going down the driveway. Even though it was through the woods, snow had accumulated to about two feet deep. I had a large flashlight with me which gave the woods, filled with howling wind and blowing snow, quite a surreal look. When I finally reached the end of the driveway by the main road the snowfall had accumulated to about four feet deep with drifts even higher. I had a little shed out there which I'd built so my kids could wait for the school bus out of the elements and, thankfully, I got to it and out of the storm. I didn't have to wait long before I saw the flashing lights of a big Caterpillar plow coming my way—the kind with a huge road plow and a wing blade that can be dropped to plow the shoulder.

The vehicle pulled up in front of me and I saw the driver motion to climb in. When I hustled up the side of the rig and into the cab I was greeted by a fellow I knew and had anesthetized about a year before, what a treat. The cab was small but had a jump seat behind the driver, and from up in the air with his floodlights on we had quite a view of the road ahead. He went down to a crossroad to get us turned around and we headed for town.

He said, "Ron, I hope it's not a life-or-death emergency, because I'd sure like to plow this stretch on the way in."

I said, "Absolutely not, it's for an appendix so go ahead. I'd like to see how this works."

He dropped the plow and the wing, and off we went. It was noisy between the diesel engine and the scraping of the road but I was surprised at how fast we moved. My friend explained that the faster we went the farther it threw the snow. The highway to town was sparsely populated and all the country folks had a mailbox out on the road's shoulder which was right in the path of the wing blade. My friend had driven this stretch many times and knew where they all were. So, as we approached a mailbox he'd pull a lever and the hydraulics would lift the wing up and over the mailbox and then he'd drop it down again.

"Wow," I said. "That must have taken a lot of practice."

He replied, "You can't even imagine how many mailboxes I wiped out learning how to do this job. I think everybody in the county has had it happen to theirs a time or two."

He was right—I'd replaced one in the past for just that reason. We were moving along at a decent clip, throwing snow everywhere, and because there were no other vehicles on the road we made good time getting to town. I mentioned to my friend that it would be fun to do his job on a regular basis, but he said, "Up all night plowing out in the country in the winter about three to four days per week gets real old after a while. And then if the storm lasts a long time, you might be plowing all day too. Once, in the middle of the night, I accidentally hit a mailbox that was sitting on an eight-inch pipe welded to a buried wheel rim and filled with concrete. It broke the wing so badly that I couldn't move, and a crew had to come out and remove it so I could get back to town. You're better off where you are Ron."

We finally made it to the edge of town and the sanding trucks had been out so it was a pretty easy drive to the hospital.

I did the case, which finished up around midnight, and the storm was still raging so I decided to just stay at the hospital for the night. Early the next morning it was still snowing and I called the sheriff again to see about a ride home. The friendly dispatcher told me that all the plows were way out in the country so it wouldn't be possible to do that. She said, "Besides, if you're on call and at home, what's to prevent you from getting called again and us having to pull another plow to come for you? Better you stay there until the storm is over."

She had a good point. So I was at the hospital napping all day and night Saturday, reading old medical journals, eating cafeteria food, looking out the window, and starting a few IVs. It wasn't until Sunday morning that a friend of mine with a four-wheel-drive truck came to get me. By then, the storm had passed, most of the roads were open, my driveway had been plowed, and my adventure was over.

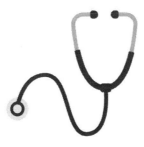

32. Janie

In the mid-'70s, there was a lady in our little North Country town (whom I'll call Janie), who could be seen most days downtown walking slightly bent over with a neck collar on. Her husband, Duane, trailed a couple of steps behind her. She was sixty-seven years old, quite thin, and always had a morose expression on her face and grayish cast to her complexion.

Janie had a ritual that all the hospital ER nurses were quite familiar with. Every Friday she would present herself to the emergency room complaining of left breast pain. Janie would be admitted to the ER and the doctor on call notified, whereupon he would order a shot of Demerol for her. It made her sleepy for a couple hours, and after a nap, Duane would take her home. According to one of the nursing supervisors, this had been going on for years and evidently she had never been worked up to find the cause of her left breast pain. Janie was thought by the medical staff and townsfolk to be a classic hypochondriac.

I got to know Janie and Duane pretty well over the years due to all her Friday visits and occasionally, on days when I'd be working after-hours, I'd go see them. Many times, Janie would be awake so we could all have a little conversation, which usually centered on the reason she was in the ER. She was a pleasant lady but very seldom smiled and always appeared uncomfortable. Duane doted on her and was such a sweet and consoling guy, never leaving her side and usually holding her hand.

One Friday evening a case of mine had been delayed, so I decided to go to the ER and see Janie. I asked the nurse at the desk if she was there. "Oh, yes," she replied "Down there in her usual spot. I just gave her some Demerol about a minute ago."

I went down to Janie's cubicle and peeked in. There she was with her husband and Janie was lying quietly on the bed with Duane holding her hand. I noticed that Janie had a little bit of a darker complexion than I was used to seeing. I walked in, greeted Duane, and went over to greet Janie. She didn't answer, nor did she seem to be breathing. I casually reached over to take Janie's pulse at her wrist. There *wasn't one*! I quickly felt for a carotid pulse. That was absent too. I asked Duane to please step out to the waiting room for a minute so I could examine her, which he did.

Once the ER door shut behind him I yelled for the nurse to bring the crash cart in and call a code blue to the ER and I immediately started chest compressions. Everybody came running to the cubicle. The nurse hooked her up to the EKG monitor and handed me an AMBU bag so I could ventilate her with 100 percent oxygen, and took over the compressions while another nurse tried to start an IV. We stopped for a couple seconds, and her EKG was flat lined. By then the on-call doctor had arrived and I quickly brought him up to speed. The nurse had been lucky enough to get an IV in Janie and the doctor immediately gave her some epinephrine. After another minute we stopped compressions again. Her EKG was still flat lined. We started CPR again, giving her more epinephrine, ventilating her, and doing chest compressions. This went on for a while, but we could not get Janie's heart started. Finally, after about forty-five minutes, the doctor called it off and pronounced her dead.

We cleaned Janie up and moved her to a private room where Duane could be with her. The poor man was so distraught he could barely speak between sobs. He and Janie had been married for over forty years and were inseparable. He told us they had no family in town, so we all stayed with him until the mortuary arrived. It really cast a pall over the ER staff afterward. Everybody knew and loved Janie and empathized with her suffering.

Epilogue:

As I mentioned, Janie had never been worked up to determine the cause of her left breast pain. In his grief Duane wanted Janie to have an autopsy to find out what her problem(s) were. About two weeks later, the results came back which corresponded completely with her symptoms. The pain was not from her left breast at all. Janie had severe coronary artery disease, with one of her coronary arteries completely occluded. The pain she experienced was from angina due to an insufficient blood supply to her heart. Janie had suffered a massive heart attack lying there in the ER and had probably died almost immediately. Duane didn't notice it because she was always very quiet in the hospital, and her skin color wasn't much different than usual.

You can never take anything for granted...

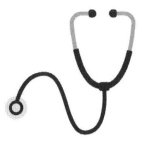

33. The Horse Bite

On a Saturday in the early '70s, while my partner was out of town, I was on call and not feeling well. Mid-morning, the hospital called to tell me that I had to come in for a little girl who had been bitten in the face by a horse and needed her lacerations repaired. A child with a probable full stomach needing emergency facial surgery is a daunting case, so I had a lot to consider on my drive in.

When I arrived, I went to the emergency room to see the little girl and make a preoperative assessment. To my amazement, she was the five-year-old daughter of some good friends and I knew the little girl well, which was a gift. At least I knew she might be cooperative with me. The family owned a large farm east of town with four horses on it: three geldings and a mare. Evidently, while in the pasture, the little girl got between the mare and her favorite gelding and the mare got feisty and bit her in the face, lifting her off the ground in the process. The girl's screaming scared the horses off, which probably saved her from more serious injuries.

When I saw the family in the ER, she was sitting on her mom's lap sniffling a little with a large gauze dressing on her left cheek. That was a big relief: her injury didn't involve her eyes, nose, or mouth. Another bit of good news was that she only had a small glass of orange juice to drink that morning because she was in such a hurry to get outside and see the horses. We had a short discussion about me giving her a little "mosquito bite" in her hand just before she went to sleep, along with "blowing up a balloon." Sweet little girl that she was, she said that would be okay.

When we had her in the OR, I gave her the "little mosquito bite" IV and she blew up the "balloon" of 100 percent oxygen for a minute or two. I injected sodium pentothal and muscle relaxant into her IV, quickly put a breathing tube in her airway, and turned on the inhalation anesthetic. After she was asleep, we took the gauze dressing off her face and saw two superficial lacerations and one deep laceration about three inches long, which looked like it might have penetrated the cheek into her mouth. The plastic repair on those lacerations—done with small, almost hair-like sutures—was slow-going.

In those days, we didn't have gas evacuators on our anesthesia machines, just a three-foot hose from the exhaust valve that blew all expired gasses into the OR. The inhalation anesthetic of choice in those days, along with nitrous oxide and oxygen, was halothane which is a halogenated hydrocarbon that has a semisweet odor to it. There was always a hint of it in the air during a case but it was more pronounced closer to the anesthesia machine.

As I mentioned earlier, I wasn't feeling well that day and occasional whiffs of that sweet Halothane smell were making me queasy. About two hours into the case I was so nauseated that I called my circulating nurse over and told her that she'd have to take over the anesthesia for a bit because I was sick to my stomach and needed to get to the bathroom right away. She was an experienced OR nurse who had been around anesthesia providers for years and stepped right up to the machine and took over.

I rushed out of the OR to the nearest bathroom—in the women's locker room—and had to stay there for a while. When I finally felt better and headed back to the OR, I thought I heard crying. As I entered, there was my little patient lying on her side with the breathing tube out, breathing just fine on her own, dressings on her face, moving all her extremities and making the little whimpering noises that I'd heard. I was amazed. Not only had the circulating nurse kept our little girl asleep until the end of the case, she had also taken her through the emergence phase to wide awake, which is one of the most critical times of an anesthetic. It couldn't have been a better ending to the case. We took our patient to the recovery room and into the waiting arms of her mother.

I thanked my circulator profusely and recommended that she apply to anesthesia school.

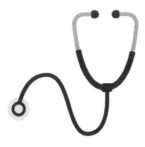

34. Anesthesia Allergy

Before my partner and I arrived at the little hospital in northern Minnesota, two brothers who had worked there for years had provided all the anesthesia. They were registered nurses, trained in a hospital by a CRNA however they had never taken the National Board exam and were not certified nurse anesthetists. From the looks of the department when we took over, it was pretty obvious that they hadn't kept current on the techniques and therapeutics of 1970s anesthesia practice.

I was asked to review an anesthesia record from the '60s regarding a ruptured spleen case one of the brothers had done, in which an otherwise healthy sixteen-year-old boy died on the operating table right after the surgery was finished. His family had been told that he was allergic to the anesthetic and that was why he died and evidently they accepted that explanation. The reason they wanted me to look at the record was because another member of the family was going to have surgery soon and they were concerned about a possible genetic familial allergy and that the same anesthetic might be used, causing another death. I was happy to do the review for them, even though their story didn't sound plausible.

When I obtained the ten-year-old chart, it didn't take much studying to realize what had happened. The young boy had just left a pizza parlor and was involved in a bad auto accident during which he'd been thrown against the dashboard and ruptured his spleen. An injury of that sort can cause massive internal bleeding and needs immediate surgery to remove the spleen and control the bleed. He was brought to the hospital in a timely fashion and was prepped for surgery with two large bore IVs.

The record showed that the patient had apparently been anesthetized for the two-hour case without the use of a breathing (endotracheal) tube to seal off his airway from possible regurgitation and aspiration of his stomach's partially digested pizza contents. The anesthetist had only used a face mask to ventilate him for the duration of the case, leaving his airway completely unsecured and unprotected. Consequently, at the end of surgery during the emergence from anesthesia, the young boy vomited a massive amount of undigested pizza into his airway that couldn't be cleared, aspirated it into his lungs and he died. I was shocked because that was a complete breach of technique for the handling of patients in those situations. Airway management and protection is one of the cardinal rules of all anesthesia practice.

I was in a bit of a quandary as to what I should say, since I knew the folks well and the incident had happened ten years prior. Granted, it was an egregious error but the anesthetist in question was long gone and the family had moved on. I decided to say as little as possible and still reassure everyone that their relative would be safe. I told them they needn't worry—I had reviewed the case and could assure them that we didn't employ the techniques and anesthetics that were used back then. They were relieved, and I was glad they didn't ask me more questions about it.

Epilogue:

About one week later I administered an anesthetic to the worried person, and everything turned out fine.

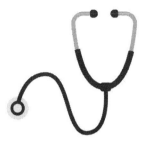

35. The Baseball Player

In 1998 I worked at a small hospital in Florida for a mixed group of twenty CRNAs and seven anesthesiologists. The CRNAs covered all the surgical cases, obstetrical cases, and labor epidurals. Labor and delivery had twelve birthing rooms and was always busy. On a late afternoon while I was covering obstetrics, one of the anesthesiologists (whom I'll call Frank) told me that the girlfriend of a very good friend of his was in early labor and would need a labor epidural at some point. He told me her name and that he had promised his friend he would be there to perform the epidural the minute she needed it. He mentioned he was leaving the hospital for a bit but asked me to call him as soon as I was notified she was ready, at which point he would come right back. I assured him I would.

About an hour went by before they called me for her epidural, and I dutifully paged Frank's beeper. He didn't respond. After about ten minutes I paged him again. Another fifteen minutes went by. Obstetrics called and said the lady was in hard labor and needed her epidural STAT! We couldn't wait any longer, so I hurried to take care of it without Frank.

Those were the days when a woman in labor could have all the people she wanted with her in the birthing room and when I arrived I was surprised to see it was full of people—all relatives of hers and her boyfriend's. I introduced myself to everyone and immediately Frank's friend asked, "Where the hell is Frank?" I had to confess that he'd left the hospital and that I'd paged him twice with no response. The lady in labor said, "I don't care where the hell Frank is, just hurry up and get rid of this damn pain."

I got all my equipment ready and got the lady sitting up on the edge of the bed facing away from me, with her boyfriend in front of her holding her in position. As I was prepping her back and locating my landmarks, I had a little conversation with the boyfriend. He said he and Frank were friends from way back in West Virginia. I asked what kind of work he did, and he told me he played baseball.

"No kidding," I replied. "Who do you play for, the Dunedin Blue Jays?"

He gave me a strange look and replied loudly, and slightly irritated, "No I play for the Yankees!"

I was about to apologize when his girlfriend asked, "Are you sure this guy is from Frank's group?"

I was embarrassed because I didn't follow baseball much then, had forgotten to ask his name, and didn't recognize him. Fortunately, I had just finished putting the lady's epidural in and dosed it and she was comfortable, which changed the entire course of our conversation. Everybody was happy, and I left to do my charting.

As I was leaving the department I ran into Frank hurrying down the hallway. He asked, "What room is she in?" I told him to calm down that I'd already put the epidural in and she was comfortable. I asked him who his friend was. He told me his name and continued with, "You're really out of it, Ron. He's one of the most famous pitchers in baseball today and has a no hitter under his belt." When I told him about my ignorant comment and how his friend had responded, Frank laughed so hard he had to sit down.

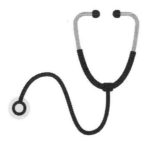

36. Dead Battery

Pulp cutters who worked in the woods surrounding our little northern Minnesota town were a tough breed, putting in long hours cutting down poplar trees for paper mills. It was tedious, messy, chainsaw work cutting, limbing, and stacking those eight-foot-long logs to be hauled off. Many of them worked fifteen-hour days year-round.

One cold fall Saturday evening in the '70s, I got a call to come to the hospital for a woods injury. They said the patient hadn't arrived yet but was en route in an ambulance from Blackduck, a small town twenty-five miles north of Bemidji. Running through my mind as I went to the hospital were all the horrible injuries that could be sustained while dealing with a pulp cutter and a chainsaw in the woods.

When I got to the emergency room, they told me the ambulance hadn't arrived yet, and they had no idea what kind of injury the patient had so I went to the OR to make sure I had everything ready for whatever I trauma I might have to deal with. After about an hour the ER still hadn't heard a word and I decided to go to the cafeteria for dinner and then back to the OR lounge to wait. Another hour went by, and the ER called me to say the police from Blackduck had just contacted them. It seems the first ambulance had some trouble so another one was dispatched to get the patient and they were finally on their way. After another hour's wait, the ambulance finally arrived and the EMT driver told us that our patient had a branch sticking out of his chest.

The surgeon and I climbed in, to find a thin, shivering fellow dressed in dirty, sawdust-covered overalls with a broken-off branch sticking out of the right side of his jacket. He tried to speak but was gasping so badly that he couldn't get many words out. His color was grayish because they hadn't even put any oxygen on him. I yelled for an O2 tank and we loaded him onto a stretcher and got him inside. The nurses covered him with warm blankets and called for a chest x-ray while I got an IV started and the surgeon carefully cut his clothes away from around the branch. Once his chest was exposed, we saw a one-inch poplar branch sticking a foot out of his right chest and about three inches lateral to his nipple. It had obviously penetrated his chest cavity, because we could hear air hissing from around the injury every time he took a breath—a classic sucking chest wound.

His color was already better from the oxygen, he was warm, his vital signs were stable, and there was no frank bleeding coming from the penetration site. So, we were fairly certain the branch hadn't done any significant internal damage. The surgeon didn't dare pull the branch out until we had the chest x-ray. When we got it, we studied the x-ray which revealed that the branch had barely entered his thoracic cavity. Probably his heavy overalls and shirt kept it from going deeper and into his lung. The surgeon pulled the branch out slowly, cleaned up the wound, put a chest tube and a few sutures in, and covered it all with sterile heavy Vaseline gauze. The head nurse called Minneapolis for their air ambulance to come get our patient, and I gave him 1 cc of Innovar IV to help him relax.

What happened to the first ambulance is a bizarre story. The two-lane road between Blackduck and Bemidji is sparsely populated and heavily wooded. After the first ambulance had picked the patient up and headed toward Bemidji, it suddenly conked out. As luck would have it, they were able to coast into the parking lot of a little roadside tavern in the woods. The ambulance's two-way radio was without power, since the vehicle wasn't working, so one of the EMT drivers had to go into the tavern and use the phone to call Blackduck and have them send another ambulance.

Seeing an EMT in the bar area generated a lot of interest from patrons, and many went outside to see what was going on. After looking in and seeing our poor patient, a few of them crawled in to offer him some whiskey to calm his nerves which, of course, was all right with the EMT. As the driver told me after we had our patient stabilized, the patient had been having trouble breathing and when the ambulance quit, it was dark and he was so cold and scared thinking he might die in the tavern parking lot, that the driver figured a couple shots couldn't hurt.

The Minneapolis team that arrived to pick him up around midnight was very happy to see that he was in better shape than they'd expected.

Two months later, we heard that he was back in the woods, pulp-cutting away...

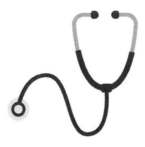

37. The Queen

Late one fall Saturday evening in the '80s, I got a call from the hospital to come in for a lady having a miscarriage and in need of an emergency dilatation and curettage. When I arrived, the patient was already in the ER lying head-down on the stretcher and looking pretty pale from blood loss. She was a young girl who had arrived by ambulance from a small town not far from Bemidji and the nurses told me that she was the homecoming queen there and that this all had happened in the middle of the ceremony.

I introduced myself to the patient and her family and during my anesthesia assessment I found out that she was otherwise healthy but had eaten a big meal that evening and drank a few beers. Fortunately, the ER nurse already had a large bore IV running in her and blood had been sent to the lab for a type and crossmatch. The gynecologist and surgical team were also there so we took her right to the operating room.

When administering emergency anesthesia to a patient with a full stomach, all things considered, the primary concern is protection of the patient's airway. Allowing gastric contents to enter a patient's airway and lungs can cause a multitude of problems, none of which are minor. The crucial time is during the induction of anesthesia—the period between when the anesthetic drugs are injected into the IV and the breathing tube is put in place in the patient's trachea with the cuff securely inflated to safely seal it off. In order to accomplish this, all anesthesia providers employ a technique called a rapid sequence induction (RSI). RSI involves administering an IV dose of Pentothal and fast-acting muscle relaxant in rapid succession while an assistant applies gentle pressure to the patient's neck, just below their Adam's apple, followed by immediate insertion of a breathing tube into the patient's trachea and inflation of the tube's circumferential balloon.

A week before this evening, a pharmaceutical representative had come to our department and introduced us to a brand-new anesthesia muscle relaxant with properties far more advantageous than the drugs we were using. The drug was associated with a small incidence of histamine release, which is a phenomenon that can cause allergic reactions. Many of our other anesthesia drugs also had that property, and I had never seen it happen. I decided to use this new drug for our case.

After our patient was on the OR table and ready to be put to sleep, I thought it would be wise to give her a very small test dose of the new drug. I drew up a miniscule amount of it (about .2 ccs) and injected it into her IV. Within a minute, red blotches began to appear all over her body and she complained of her tongue feeling swollen and shortness of breath. Her pulse was 135 beats per minute, and I couldn't get an accurate blood pressure. She was agitated to the point of jerking around on the table. I yelled for the gynecologist, who was at the scrub sink, to come help me because our patient was having an anaphylactic reaction. She was rapidly losing consciousness, so I quickly put in a breathing tube to ventilate her with 100 percent oxygen.

In the absence of a readable blood pressure, and with her pulse becoming rapid and faint, we instituted CPR. The gynecologist and scrub tech alternated doing chest compressions, and while I ventilated her, the circulating nurse drew up and administered IV steroids, Benadryl, and epinephrine. After about twenty minutes of this, I was able to get a readable blood pressure and begin to hear her pulse. She also started to wake up and object to the breathing tube. Her vital signs were stable by then, so I took the endotracheal tube out and put an oxygen mask on her. The gynecologist said that she wasn't going to do the procedure that evening after all that had happened and she wanted to wait and do it the following morning. So the doctor packed the young lady's vagina and we sent her to ICU to be observed and monitored for the night.

Bright and early the next morning, we scheduled the young girl for her procedure. She had received two units of blood during the night and looked much better than when she came into the ER. Her doctor from the evening before was not on call then; her partner would be doing the case. He said that after talking it over with the patient and reading her chart, he would prefer to do the case without her having any anesthesia drugs at all. I spoke with the young lady and her family about our plans for her procedure, and she was frightened, but she remembered just enough from the previous evening to be okay with it.

We brought her to the OR, did the short procedure, and although it was uncomfortable, she tolerated it very well and we were all relieved when it was over. Her family thanked us profusely.

I never used that drug again in all my years.

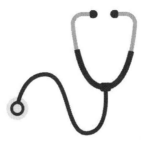

38. Helping with the AAA

In the 1970s, we had a well-trained surgeon at our little hospital who electively repaired abdominal aortic aneurysms (AAA). These are demanding cases with a lot of considerations for the whole surgical team and often took many hours to complete. We didn't have the sophisticated monitoring equipment in use today; all of our anesthetic techniques then were based on observation of the patient, our judgment, and the few rudimentary tools at our disposal. With adequate preparation, this was almost never a problem. Because there were only two CRNAs (me and my partner) in the department, it usually meant one of us would be doing the case by ourselves with only a circulating nurse to help out in the event of a crisis, while the other CRNA was doing cases in another room.

One cold winter's morning, there was an AAA repair on a relatively healthy man scheduled as the first case in my partner's room and I had a bunch of short cases in my own room. All seemed to be going well, but after my second case was finished the OR supervisor asked me to please go help my partner in the AAA room because he needed a second set of anesthesia hands to pump blood. As I rushed into the room to help him, I slipped on a small puddle of water from the scrub sink just inside the door and staggered forward, grabbing one of his IV poles to keep from falling into the surgical field. The IV pole was on wheels and the force of my forward motion pushed it, with a loud crash, into the wall six feet away. That jerked the patient's only large bore IV out of his arm!

The pole had a unit of whole blood on a pressure pump hanging from it and when the IV came out the pressure from the pump on the blood bag caused the

IV tubing to whip all over the place, squirting blood on the wall, the circulating nurse, and her charting table. Fortunately, the nurse leapt over to the IV tubing and quickly clamped it shut. It all happened so fast that my partner and I just looked at each other for a moment, then we quickly grabbed a couple of large bore IV catheters and stuck them into the patient's jugular veins on either side of his neck. By now, the OR supervisor and the circulator—who was covered with blood—had two IVs with blood sets ready to go. We hooked them up, put up a unit of blood on a pump on each one, and were able to transfuse the patient back to a normal blood pressure. The surgeon looked up unruffled and said, "Nice work, boys, but what a damn mess you made."

The rest of the case went very well, and the patient was discharged one week later.

I hope nobody ever told him what happened during his surgery.

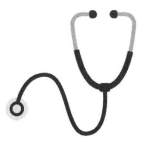

39. Motorcycle Head Injury

On a beautiful summer Saturday morning, while I was on call, I happened to be in town shopping. Since this was before beepers or cell phones were readily available, I'd call the hospital operator and tell her where I was every time I went to a different store and give her their phone number. Around mid-morning, she told me I needed to come in right away for a motorcycle accident victim who was in an ambulance en route to the ER.

When I arrived at the emergency room the ambulance had just pulled in. Our patient was a young man who had been involved in a crash out on the highway and looked to be in very bad shape. He also happened to be one of the respiratory therapists who worked at the hospital and was very well-liked by everyone. His face was smashed and bloody to the point of being unrecognizable. Where his mouth should have been was a gaping, bloody hole with bubbles and gurgling sounds coming out of it. That he was still trying to breathe through all that trauma was miraculous.

I had to get a breathing (endotracheal) tube into his airway right away for there to be any chance he might survive. While a nurse helped, suctioning the blood out of his mouth, I put the blade of my laryngoscope into it and it was like looking into an inkwell. The end of the laryngoscope blade had a bright light on it and I could just make out a few bubbles coming up from somewhere down lower. I figured they were from his trachea, so I carefully inserted the breathing tube into that mess following the stream of bubbles. When it was in to an appropriate depth and hadn't met any resistance I decided to blow up the cuff to, hopefully, seal off his airway and hook it up to a portable ventilating device (AMBU bag) and see if it was in the right place. *Success!*

Through pure luck, Divine intervention, and a measure of expertise, the tube had gone into his trachea. I attached the AMBU to 100 percent oxygen and was able to adequately breathe for him. About that time the surgeon arrived and was in a big hurry. He came storming into the ER, yelling, "Let's go! Let's go! We gotta get to surgery." Without bothering to talk to any of us who had been treating the young man, he just grabbed the foot end of the ER cart and jerked it toward the surgery doors. I turned around briefly to disconnect the oxygen tubing from the wall outlet and when I turned back, the cart and our patient were all the way down the hall and I was left standing there holding the AMBU with the bloody breathing tube attached to it that I had just struggled to put in the young man's trachea.

You should've seen the horrified looks on the faces of the ER personnel. I yelled at them to stop, but the doors had closed. I ran down the hall after the cart but by the time I got to the OR the patient had stopped making any respiratory effort. His mouth area was even a bigger mess than before, having had that tube jerked out of it, and he had no pulse or blood pressure. I struggled to get the endotracheal back into his airway, without success. After about fifteen minutes the surgeon pronounced him dead.

Epilogue:

I never mentioned anything to the surgeon about pulling the endotracheal tube out of the patient's airway by how he yanked the cart. We all (including the surgeon) knew what a bad mistake that was but in my estimation, even under the best circumstances, the young fellow probably would have died anyway from his terrible injuries.

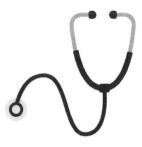

40. The Supraglottic Tumor

The hospital I worked at in Florida had many specialty surgeons doing cases in our ten-room OR. On any given day a case in my room could be a simple carpal tunnel release or a big neurosurgery and everything in between.

My first case one morning was scheduled as a biopsy and excision of a glottic mass just above the vocal cords. According to the ENT surgeon, the mass was large, quite friable (bleeds easily), and significantly protruded into the airway. My patient was a pleasant, thirty-two-year-old otherwise healthy woman who was slightly hoarse and occasionally experienced shortness of breath on exertion. The surgeon requested that my attending anesthesiologist perform the intubation, because the possibility of massive bleeding from the friable tumor could necessitate an emergency tracheotomy. I had a discussion with the patient about the possibility of her waking up with a tracheotomy tube in her neck due to the size of the tumor and she was frightened but understood and accepted it.

Tracheotomy is a surgical opening into the trachea just below the Adam's apple to bypass any form of upper airway obstruction that is not able to be quickly and easily cleared. In surgery, once that opening is made a special tube with an inflatable cuff around it is inserted to seal off the trachea and provide the patient the ability to adequately breathe or be ventilated. As you might expect in an emergency for airway patency, time is of the essence.

For the intubation of our patient, we had elected to use a fiber-optic video laryngoscope called a Glide Scope. The instrument has a video camera and a very bright light at the end of the laryngoscope blade that projects a clear image of the oral cavity and airway onto an eight-inch screen placed right next to the patient's head. A Glide Scope is generally used for all critical and difficult intubations.

After our patient was anesthetized, relaxed and easy to ventilate, my attending anesthesiologist gingerly inserted the blade of the Glide Scope into her mouth. We visualized her airway and it was quite an intimidating sight. The tumor was a round, grayish, blood-streaked mass protruding halfway into the opening to her trachea and immediately above the vocal cords. I cautioned my attending to be extremely careful not to touch the tumor with his endotracheal tube until it was in the partial opening to the trachea and then to quickly advance it and inflate the cuff to seal off the airway from bleeding that was sure to occur.

My exact words were, "Make damn sure you don't touch that tumor until the tube is in the trachea, because if we get a lot of bleeding and have to do an emergency trach, we're in real trouble! This surgeon is the slowest guy on the planet and he can't do anything fast. I did a trach with him once that took almost an hour and, thank Heaven, it wasn't an emergency, or the patient might not have made it."

My attending slowly inserted the endotracheal tube, and as it approached the small opening into the trachea, he inadvertently scraped the side of the tumor. Immediately, it started to gush blood! He pulled the tube and laryngoscope out of her mouth, and I yelled for the surgeon—who was at the scrub sink—to get in the room and get an emergency tracheotomy into our patient ASAP! I grabbed a suction handle (Yankauer) and was able to suck blood out as fast as it was welling up and got the mask attached to the anesthesia circuit on her face to try to ventilate her. Surprisingly, I could move a little oxygen into her as long as my attending was there to suck blood out of her mouth as I did it. I had enough of a ventilatory exchange to keep her oxygen saturation at 88 to 92 percent; it was a bloody mess though.

Every time I got a breath into her, she exhaled it with a blood splatter into the mask. The ENT surgeon came into the room, obviously annoyed that all this was happening. He wasn't moving fast and was making demands for the instruments he wanted. I told him, "Hurry up and get a trach in this lady, because I don't know how long this bloody airway will hold out." He glared at me, finished drying his hands, and walked over to the OR table.

From the time he started doing the emergency tracheotomy until he finished, and the lady had a patent airway, was fifty-five minutes. In all my years of anesthesia I've never worked with another surgeon who took that long to perform an emergency tracheotomy. It was pure agony watching the surgeon work and do a slow, overly methodical dissection in the patient's neck to get down to her trachea. All the while, he complained about the lack of exposure while my attending and I were suctioning the blood spewing out of her mouth, trying to ventilate her adequately, and periodically wiping the gore off her face. Thank Heaven we had put ophthalmic ointment in her eyes and taped them shut.

Every time we mentioned hurrying, he gave us an annoyed look. At last he popped the tracheotomy tube into her neck, blew up the cuff, and I could hook the anesthesia circuit up to it and ventilate her adequately. What a relief to all of us! The head of the table was a bloody mess, so we cleaned the patient's face and re-draped everything so we could finally start the case. Fortunately, throughout the whole fifty-five-minute tracheotomy fiasco, the patient's vital signs remained stable and her oxygen saturation never dropped below 88 percent. We called it a miracle!

The rest of the case went well. It took another hour and one half for the methodical surgeon to resect the airway tumor and control the bleeding, but at the end of the case, all was well. We took our patient to the recovery room in stable condition, where she woke up just fine.

My attending and I had a long discussion about that case, and we put it on the agenda for our next department meeting.

A month later our anesthesia department met and I presented the case. After many surprised looks and a lot of gasps, my attending and I fielded questions about the circumstances surrounding it. The general consensus was that there was probably a slim chance the patient's airway could've been intubated without a massive bleed occurring and that we should've had the surgeon in the room with all his instruments ready to go for an emergency tracheotomy while we did it. Everybody agreed, however, that the biggest threat to the patient's well being was the fact that the surgeon took fifty-five minutes to get the tracheotomy tube in place which could've been disastrous had we not been able to ventilate her at all. Fortunately, there were other surgeons in the department that probably could've come into our OR and accomplished the procedure in minutes. I'm glad we never had to call them but it was resolved that if a CRNA was ever involved in a similar situation, with that particular doctor, to call their attending MDA and another surgeon immediately.

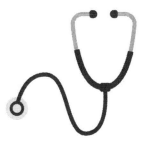

41. The Specimen Jar

In 1975 there were only the two of us CRNAs to handle all the anesthesia needs in our little three-room OR suite in northern Minnesota. Whoever was on call worked in the room that had the most number of cases in it and would finish up last.

One morning I was doing gynecology cases with our OB/GYN doctor. My first case was scheduled as a dilatation and curettage (D and C). The patient was a pleasant lady in her mid-thirties, in good health, and whose preop diagnosis was menorrhagia. A dilatation and curettage is a relatively short procedure that involves dilating the cervix and scraping out the inside of the uterus with an instrument called a curette. Once I had the patient adequately anesthetized and spontaneously breathing anesthetic gasses, I gave the surgeon permission to start the procedure.

As he was working, I noticed that I didn't have all my anesthesia papers and, because the circulating nurse was busy, I briefly stepped to the back table where the patient's chart was located. I noticed a specimen jar sitting on the table next to the chart, so I casually picked it up and held it up to the light to see what was in it. To my horror, floating in the formalin was a perfectly formed little fetus about a half-inch long and with the light coming through it, I could see its little heart beating. I immediately put the jar down, got a queasy stomach, and hustled back to the head of the table with my papers. I never said a word about it to anyone in the OR, but I'm pretty sure some of the old-timers there knew what was going on. I was conflicted after that because with only the two of us to do all the anesthesia I really had no choice but to continue doing those kinds of cases for that doctor. As it turns out, about a year later he had a massive heart attack and died. The OB/GYN doctor who replaced him from Minneapolis didn't do those kinds of procedures.

I was only thirty-five at the time, and until then hadn't really developed any particular feelings about abortion.

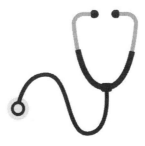

42. Innovar Hypo

In the late '60s, a new drug was introduced to the anesthesia world called Innovar. It was a combination of two drugs: fentanyl and droperidol. When administered intravenously, in conjunction with light inhalation anesthetic agents, it produced profound analgesia (pain control) and a detachment from external stimuli with a phenomenon called neuroleptanalgesia. It was also an excellent preoperative medication that could be administered intramuscularly to put the patient into a very relaxed, drowsy state.

Fentanyl is a synthetic narcotic more potent than morphine and droperidol and has anti-nausea and mild sedative effects. In pharmacology literature, dysphoria (anxiety, restlessness, unease, dissatisfaction, paranoia) is listed as an uncommon side effect from droperidol. I used Innovar frequently because it provided such a wonderful adjunct to our anesthetic techniques in that it decreased the dosages needed for most of the other agents.

One cold winter morning, for my second case that day, I had a middle-aged man (whom I'll call Roger) as a patient for an inguinal hernia repair. He arrived at the hospital alone—his wife planned to come after she was done working. He was a healthy and quite active fellow, and after my interview with him I wrote an order for 2 ccs of Innovar IM (intramuscularly) as his preop hypo on call to the OR. Halfway through my first case I sent word to give Roger his preop hypo. I took my patient to the recovery room, got set up for Roger's case, and our team went for a short break.

While we were having coffee, the head nurse from preop came in and said that they'd given Roger his hypo about an hour earlier and now they couldn't find him. According to the nurse, his clothes and hospital gown were still in the room. They'd looked everywhere, but he was nowhere to be found. The nursing supervisor had been alerted, and everybody in the hospital who wasn't occupied was looking for him. A half hour later, the maintenance department called us to say they had located Roger. A visitor had noticed a car running in the parking lot with a man sitting in the driver's seat who didn't appear to be wearing clothes. A bunch of staff members went to check. Sure enough, it was Roger.

As they approached the car, Roger cracked open the window and warned them not to come any closer, because he had a gun and wasn't going to be taken alive. I told them to call Roger's wife right away and ran outside to see if I could reason with him. As I approached the car, Roger warned me off. I asked him if he remembered our talk about his hernia surgery earlier. He said yes but that I was just as bad as the rest of them. He never told us what he was afraid of but just kept repeating that we were bad and that he didn't trust us. It was impossible to reason with him no matter what we said. When I told him that his wife was on the way, he scoffed at that and said that she couldn't change his mind about "what he knew was going on." I told him that he needed to have clothes on because it was winter. His reply: "That stuff you put on me was all wired. I know your game."

Finally Roger's wife arrived, visibly upset and crying. Before she approached his car, I took her aside and explained to her that I was pretty sure Roger was having a rare side effect of one of the drugs he'd had in his preop hypo and that it was only a matter of time until it wore off and he'd be his normal self again. I told her not to be surprised or offended by anything he said, because it was the drug talking, not him. When she approached his car and implored him to stop what he was doing, he told her that she was just in cahoots with us and to quit listening to what we said.

While she kept a steady conversation going with Roger, I had a meeting with the nursing staff and maintenance fellows out in the parking lot. We decided that at least three people, one of whom was a nurse, had to be by his car with him and his wife at all times until he calmed down and listened to reason, and they also needed to have some warm clothes for him when he calmed down. We also called the police department to explain the situation and had them send a cruiser over to be in the parking lot where Roger could see it.

I had other cases to do, so I went back to the OR and got periodic reports on Roger's situation. He seemed to be content just sitting in his car with the engine running, and the staff assigned to watch him switched out every half hour. Occasionally, his wife would go inside to warm up. Finally, after about three hours of this, Roger started to listen to reason. He admitted to his wife that he didn't know why he was out in his car and let the hospital staff get him clothed and into a warm coat. What a relief! We got Roger back to the preop department, restarted his IV, and by the middle of the afternoon fixed his hernia. After he was anesthetized, I gave him a mild tranquilizer, hoping it might dull his memory of the episode and let him wake up comfortably.

Epilogue:

Roger's surgery and recovery period were uneventful, and not a word was mentioned about the morning's chaos.

I never used Innovar for a preop hypo again.

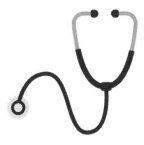

43. Two Tourniquet Stories

Xylocaine Allergy

For most lower-arm surgical cases a tourniquet is routinely used and the patient may have a general anesthetic, a local anesthetic plus intravenous sedation, or a regional anesthetic plus sedation. One very common type of regional anesthetic, for relatively short lower-arm procedures, is called a Bier block. For this type of anesthetic, a small intravenous catheter is placed in the patient's hand on the affected side, the area where the tourniquet is to be applied on the upper arm is wrapped with padding, and the tourniquet is placed over it. The lower arm is then wrapped with an elastic bandage up to the tourniquet to squeeze all the blood out of it. Once the arm is exsanguinated, the tourniquet is inflated to 250 mm of mercury, and a 50 cc solution of .25-percent xylocaine is injected through the intravenous catheter in the patient's hand to effectively fill the whole arm with local anesthetic. This provides the patient with a profoundly numb arm and a bloodless field for the surgeon for up to an hour and a half, at which time the tourniquet is deflated.

If the patient is not asleep and only sedated, they may occasionally complain of tourniquet pain toward the end of the case. A relatively recent addition to this technique is the double tourniquet, one right next to the other one. After the xylocaine solution is injected into the patient's arm, the proximal tourniquet is inflated. When the patient complains of discomfort from it, the distal tourniquet is inflated and the proximal one deflated so that now the inflated tourniquet is in the numb area of the patient's arm and their discomfort is gone. For short cases, the tourniquet may be deflated after thirty minutes with no systemic effects to the patient from the local anesthetic. Bier blocks have been in use for a long time and were first discovered and administered by August Bier in 1908.

One morning, in the mid-'70s, my first patient of the day was a pretty healthy old fellow who had lived in the woods his whole life. He hadn't been to see a doctor in many years and had a log fall on his right hand, fracturing his little finger when he was chopping wood. That had been about a month prior but he hadn't seen any need to have it looked at because it didn't hurt much. His finger healed at a thirty-degree angle and was getting in his way so he had finally decided to have it fixed. When I asked him if he had allergies, especially to medications, he said he didn't take pills but that he might have been allergic to something thirty years ago, though he had no idea what it was or what the circumstances were. I explained everything to him about a Bier block anesthetic for his arm, and he agreed that it would be fine.

After I got his IV started, and gave him a small dose of tranquilizer, I got him all set up for the block. I wrapped his arm in an elastic bandage, put up the tourniquet, and injected my xylocaine solution through the IV catheter in his hand. Immediately his whole arm up to the tourniquet turned a bright cherry red! At that moment I was positive I knew what he'd been allergic to thirty years ago: lidocaine. Thank Heaven the tourniquet was up so he didn't get it systemically!

I explained to him what had just happened and called for the surgeon. Even though the incidence of allergy to lidocaine is pretty low, we discussed it and canceled the case. I got on the phone to the University of Minnesota Hospital anesthesia department right away and explained our situation. The chief resident there was very helpful and told me to first load the patient up with steroids, give him a dose of Benadryl, and after one hour let the tourniquet down for two seconds, increasing the time by one second every half hour for three hours. If the patient showed no signs of an allergic reaction after the last time we let it down to leave it down but admit him to ICU for observation for twenty-four hours and be prepared at a moment's notice to treat anaphylaxis. That's exactly what we did.

I followed the chief resident's protocol and gave the patient a big dose of steroids and Benadryl, and for the next three hours sat with him in the recovery room, letting the tourniquet down for a few seconds every half hour. Thankfully, at the end, when the tourniquet was down for good, our patient didn't have an allergic reaction—but his arm stayed red. We admitted him to ICU and the next morning all was well but his arm was still red. He had full function and sensation in it and we discharged him with his red arm and bent finger later that day. I used to see him downtown occasionally after that, and over the next month his arm redness gradually decreased to just a bunch of red dots, and by the end of the summer they were gone too.

He hadn't come back to get his finger fixed by the time I left town in 1987. For all I know, it's still bent.

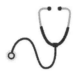

Failed Double Tourniquet

There are many therapeutic uses and side effects of intravenous lidocaine administration and when employing the Bier block technique of regional anesthesia, it's important to be aware of all of them. Two early symptoms of a lidocaine overdose are seizure activity and dysphonia. As I described in the previous Bier block episode, the double tourniquet technique is now pretty much the standard of care for this type of anesthesia.

We got our first self-contained double tourniquet set up in Bemidji in the early '80s. It was a pole-mounted electronic insufflator with outlets on it for two tourniquet hoses (hose A and hose B) to be attached. The tourniquet was a single unit with two bladders, so it didn't take up much space on the arm and was easy to apply, thereby much more convenient than managing two completely separate setups.

One morning my first case was to be a carpal tunnel release on a fellow named Vern—a good friend of mine. He had opted to have a Bier block with sedation as his anesthetic. The circulating nurse I was working with was part-time; it was her first experience working with the new double tourniquet so I carefully explained and showed her how it worked. After we got my friend on the OR table I gave him some intravenous sedation, put the new tourniquet on his arm and wrapped it with an elastic bandage to get it exsanguinated.

When it was all wrapped, I told her to inflate tourniquet A. I heard it inflate, unwrapped the arm, and injected my xylocaine solution.

As soon as I finished injecting, the circulator said, "Oops. I think I accidentally inflated tourniquet B," whereupon she deflated tourniquet B and fumbled around before finding the button for tourniquet A. Horror of horrors! I had just injected my friend's arm with 50 cc of .25 percent lidocaine and had no idea how much of it got loose into his circulation! In a loud voice I immediately asked Vern how he was doing. He answered in such a garbled voice I couldn't understand him. He sounded like a person who was extremely intoxicated, presumably due to the big dose of systemic lidocaine he'd just received.

The next possible effect could be a grand mal seizure, so I snatched up a sodium pentothal syringe and quickly injected it into the IV running in his other arm. Thankfully, Vern went to sleep before anything bad happened. I explained the situation to our surgeon and we decided that as long as he was anesthetized, we might as well go ahead with his carpal tunnel surgery and I'd monitor him closely for any possible cardiac issues. The surgery took forty-five minutes. Twenty-five minutes before it started was when Vern got the dose of xylocaine into his circulation, so we decided that any possible toxicity or side effects from it was very low. Vern's vital signs had been stable all through the procedure so when the dressings were on, with trepidation, I released the tourniquet.

What a wonderful emergence from general anesthesia Vern had. He didn't have a seizure, spoke normally, and his vital signs were still stable. I was so happy and—needless to say—so was the circulating nurse. In the recovery room Vern did well, and after a couple hours of observation, we let his wife take him home. We explained to her what had happened and that he didn't seem to have any ill effects but that she should call immediately if she or he noticed anything worrisome.

We never got a call, but a couple weeks later I happened to see Vern downtown and asked him how he was. He said his hand was healing up fine, but for a week after the surgery he had a constant buzzing in his ears.

After that experience, whenever I gave anybody a Bier block I inflated the tourniquets myself.

Lesson learned.

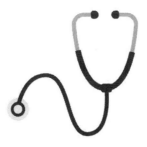

44. The Prep

Back in the '70s, standard operating procedure mandated that all patients having surgery were to be admitted to the hospital the night before. The preop prep procedure then was a body shave from nipples to knees around the area where the surgery was going to be performed. If they were the first case of the day, that shave would be very early in the morning and later cases got their shave as the day progressed.

My third case one morning was going to be a hemorrhoidectomy on a very big and hairy young fellow. He was so hairy all over his body that he practically appeared to be wearing a shaggy sweater. As we started my first case, I told them to call out to the ward and have the hemorrhoid patient prepped. In about two hours, we finished the first two cases and sent for our third one. After twenty minutes, when the patient hadn't arrived, I called the ward and asked what the holdup was. The head nurse said that her orderly was training a new fellow and it was just taking a little more time than usual to prep the patient, so I told her to call us when they were ready.

Another hour went by, and we hadn't received word. I called the ward again. The head nurse said it was taking a lot longer than usual because the patient was so hairy and that they had used four prep kits already. Finally, after another twenty minutes, the patient was ready to come to the OR. He was kind of a stoic guy, very cooperative but not much to say. Per standard procedure for a hemorrhoidectomy case, we put the patient to sleep on the OR cart, I put an endotracheal breathing tube into his airway, and then we rolled him over to the OR table on his belly.

After our fellow was anesthetized and his cover sheet and gown were removed, we were amazed to see that he was shaved clean from nipples to knees on his front side. What a sight that was! All the dense hair was gone. Obviously, the orderlies got carried away, since that wasn't the operative side of his body. We turned him over to the OR table and, lo and behold, his backside was clean as a whistle too from his shoulder blades to the back of his knees. That gave us all a good laugh trying to imagine what the poor guy must've gone through, thinking this was the way we did things. And, above those shaved areas there was still a forest of dense black hair.

When the circulator spread his buttocks to start the surgical prep, the only area that hadn't been shaved was right around his anus: the operative site. It was just as hairy as the rest of his body. Everybody in the room roared with laughter, so much so that the OR supervisor had to come in and see what was going on. The circulator shaved the site clean and we got his operation started and when it was over and we were in the recovery room, I called the head nurse on the ward and told her about the "extensive" prep. She laughed too and said she'd make sure to correct the orderlies about that in the future.

I saw the fellow around town occasionally after that and thought what a nightmare it must have been for him as all that hair grew back, but I never dared to ask him.

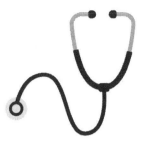

45. New Anesthesia Machine

In 1971, when I first arrived at the little northern Minnesota hospital (where I would work for sixteen years), the anesthesia department used some pretty old-fashioned equipment. It didn't have the latest cutting-edge stuff I was used to in Minneapolis. My partner and I made it work well for our anesthesia needs though, and gradually replaced and upgraded things piecemeal—everything, that is, except the anesthesia machines. Those machines, we joked, were probably from the Second World War. They were small, had old-style gauges and gas flow meters, and even had old ether jars which we never used. Finally, after a supporting arm broke on one of them, forcing us to cobble it back together, it was time to consider a replacement. My partner and I did some research and found a state-of-the art machine that was perfect for our needs. The cost: $3,200. We drew straws, and I was elected to approach administration about it.

A year after my arrival there, the hospital had hired a new administrator from southern Minnesota. I didn't know him very well, so it was with a certain amount of uneasiness that I approached the issue one morning in his office. After describing our old anesthesia machines to him and the recent situation with the supporting arm, I laid out all the research we'd done on the new machine we needed.

He looked it over pensively. "Awful expensive, don't you think?" he concluded. I replied that it wasn't the most expensive machine on the market but was absolutely perfect for our needs. He said, "That's too expensive, and I don't think we can afford it."

Now I was getting slightly annoyed. I viewed the machine as an absolute necessity, in light of the old relics we were using. So I added, "Well, we really need it, because if one of those old dogs we're using breaks in the middle of a case, it could jeopardize a patient. And besides, every one of the office personnel has the latest expensive electronic typewriter and adding machine on their desk, so what's the big deal?"

His response was classic: "Yeah, and do you know what those typewriters and adding machines on those desks do? They generate revenue!" He followed it up with, "We have to make money to pay for those big-dollar salaries you two are making."

Now I was red-hot mad! I composed myself a bit before going on, "Is that so! I'll show you firsthand what our big-dollar salaries are for! The next time I get a carload of drunks from a wreck on the highway that're all busted up and bleeding in the middle of the night, I'll give you a call to come in and help me pump blood and clean up all the cheap whiskey puke that's everywhere. And you can go talk to the family about why one of them didn't make it, because our hospital uses inferior quality anesthesia machines," I said. With that, I stomped off, leaving all the literature on his desk. He didn't say a word.

Of course, I went back to surgery and told all the staff and surgeons present about my exchange, which really surprised them. I was also good friends with the chairman of the hospital board, whom I happened to encounter at lunch that day and I had a nice chat with him about my morning encounter with our new administrator. He was visibly upset over how I'd been treated and assured me he'd get to the bottom of it. (He was the one who'd hired me and determined what my "big-dollar" salary would be...)

One week later, my partner and I received a note from the purchasing director to meet with him about ordering a new anesthesia machine. We had no more run-ins with the administrator and were superficially nice to each other in passing from then on.

These days, anesthesia machines cost between $50,000 and $150,000.

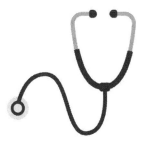

46. Crazy Days

One lovely summer morning in June, I received a call from ICU to come in right away and intubate a patient who was experiencing increasingly severe respiratory distress. This is a "hurry up and get there" kind of emergency. I lived twelve miles outside of town, so I got into my car and raced in as fast as I dared. The hospital was located in the center of downtown and a local merchant extravaganza happened to be taking place that day, so traffic was heavy.

While weaving my way through town as fast as I could, I suddenly noticed the flashing lights of a highway patrol car behind me. I had no time to stop for explanations with the trooper, so I continued weaving in and out of traffic all the way to the hospital. When I arrived, I parked right in front in the designated medical staff spot and started to run into the building. All of a sudden a hand grabbed my shoulder and spun me around, nearly making me fall. It was the trooper.

I said, "What the hell did you do that for?"

He replied, "Don't you know it's Crazy Days in town? And you were speeding and weaving in and out of traffic."

I said, "Well, in case you hadn't noticed where I parked, I have an emergency to attend to in ICU where a patient is having respiratory distress. And I don't have time to stand here and argue with you. Also, maybe you could think a little bit and figure out from the scenario that there might be something life-threatening going on here. This is a hospital, you know, and you could possibly help out instead of manhandling me. Didn't you take an oath to protect and serve? If you want to know who I am, run my plate. Maybe I should call your commandant so he can re-train you?" With that, I ran off to ICU.

I never heard a word from the highway patrol or any other law enforcement official after that. I intubated the patient and put him on the ventilator. He was much happier, and I went home.

All's well that ends well.

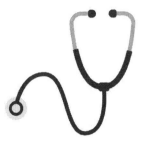

47. The Housekeeper

According to several articles I've read in hospital trade magazines, the hospital housekeeping staff generally has excellent departmental rapport and is very well-liked by inpatients. Oftentimes the same housekeeping person sees the patient five to six days a week in a nonmedical capacity and often having nice, lighthearted conversations with them as they clean the room.

One morning I was sitting outside of a room in the ICU of St. Anthony's Hospital in St. Petersburg, Florida waiting to do anesthesia for an endoscopic procedure on a patient too critical to be moved to the endoscopy department. The rooms there all had glass fronts so that patients could be observed from the hallway. I could see in the room across from mine an old man who had a lot of intravenous fluids running through a myriad of attached IV pumps and lines. An oxygen cannula was in his nose; he appeared to have slightly labored breathing as he watched TV while sitting up.

As I watched him, the housekeeper—an older African American woman—entered his room, which put a big smile on his face. The door was open, so I could hear her greet him with, "Hi, handsome. You sure look good today." She walked over to him and gave him a big hug and kiss on the forehead. Then she sat down right next to his bed, held his hand, and they had a nice conversation for about ten minutes. They kept up a running conversation throughout the entire time she spent cleaning his room, during which he smiled and even laughed a bit. Finally, when she was done she fluffed up his pillow, fixed his covers, kissed his forehead again, hugged him again, and said, "Bye, I'll see you again tomorrow, boyfriend." That old man was still smiling when the doctor arrived ten minutes later to do my case.

What a pleasant scene I had just witnessed. When I mentioned it to the ICU nurses, they told me that all the housekeepers working in ICU were like that and could sometimes become quite attached to the patients.

I told everybody in the OR about it when I got back, even going so far as to call the head of housekeeping to express my gratitude about what I had seen. Not surprisingly, she told me that she heard such positive comments frequently from patients, visitors, and the medical staff.

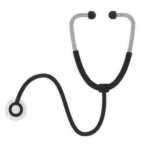

48. Incarcerated Hernia

I got a call one spring evening in the early '70s to come to the hospital for an emergency incarcerated inguinal hernia surgery. This is caused when a portion of bowel herniates through a weakened portion of groin musculature. If the bowel gets trapped there and loses its blood supply, major surgery and a bowel resection might be required to fix things. Diagnosed early enough, the hernia can be repaired and that portion of bowel returned to the patient's abdomen intact.

My patient that evening was an eighty-five-year-old bachelor farmer who lived back in the woods not far from me. He was rather reclusive, residing in a small cement block house with a coal stove for heat in the winter. Occasionally, I'd see him driving his beat-up pickup to town. He had presented himself to the ER that evening because he was having severe groin pain, which he'd had for a day or so. When I saw him in the ER, the surgeon had already examined him, determined that he had an incarcerated inguinal hernia, and wanted to take him to the OR as soon as we were ready. The only problem: The staff couldn't get his long underwear off. He had on a union suit—a one-piece suit of long underwear that buttons up the front, has a trapdoor in the back, and was made out of wool. In this old fellow's case, it was heavy wool, and he only changed it once a year—and that was during midsummer. He had worn this suit for almost nine months and, from not bathing, it was literally stuck to him! The material was well-attached to his skin everywhere, and he couldn't tolerate anybody tugging on it.

After a brief meeting of the minds, the surgeon okayed us to soak him in a lukewarm, soapy tub for a while to see if that helped. The old fellow was very agreeable to that, telling me, "This will be my first bath this year." We got him into the tub, and over the course of the next forty-five minutes, six of us gently worked on that union suit, pulling and snipping fabric, until we had it off him. His skin was a bright cherry-red after all that, and his feet, which had been black as coal dust before, were finally semi-clean. Also, one of the nurses had the good sense to wash his hair, which made the old fellow look fairly presentable. When all was said and done, the bathwater was the color of dark mud.

We got him to surgery and fixed his hernia, which fortunately didn't require a bowel resection. In the recovery room the nurses rubbed lotion all over him to help that raw skin heal. When I saw him the next morning, he said, "Damn, I feel good. I'll have to come in here once a year from now on to get cleaned up and eat good."

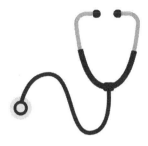

49. The Reflex

When I started anesthesia school in 1969 at the Minneapolis School of Anesthesia, my first hospital rotation was at the Hennepin County hospital. It was, and still is, a large trauma and teaching hospital. The department's chief of anesthesia then was an anesthesiologist who had many years of experience and loved to show off some of his little "tricks of the trade" to the students. His career had evolved from the old "ether dripping and chloroform" days of the '40s and '50s and he still employed many of those techniques which, according to his philosophy, "The old ways are still the best."

The induction of anesthesia period is one of the most critical times in the whole course of the anesthetic. It's the time when the patient goes from wide awake lying on the OR table to a fully anesthetized surgical state. These days, with all the beat-to-beat digital heart and blood pressure monitors, gas analyzers, and modern, fast-acting drugs in use, it's very easy to tell what status of the patient's anesthetic is in at any given time. In the '60s and '70s, it was a pure judgment—with a little guesswork mixed in—call. The patient might look and act asleep but most times, until the surgeon made a skin incision, we were never 100 percent sure. Plus, it was considered very bad technique if, when a surgeon made a skin incision, the patient moved at all.

One inexperienced student in my class had a memorable case: After the incision had been made, the patient let out a bloodcurdling scream and tried to sit up!

The old chief used a little trick to determine the depth of a patient's anesthetic right after induction. As I was preparing to start a case one day, he explained, "Ronald, if you ever get something in your eye, no matter how small, it's so stimulating that it immediately makes you blink and squint. What I'm going to show you now is a surefire way to tell if your patient is deeply anesthetized and all their reflexes are blocked."

I proceeded to give my patient a dose of sodium pentothal and muscle relaxant and, with a big sigh she drifted off to sleep. I ventilated her by mask for a few minutes, whereupon the chief stepped in to show me his "trick." He took the mask off her face, propped the lids of her left eye open with his thumb and forefinger, and with the other thumb rubbed it briskly over the cornea of that eye. Nothing happened—except my aghast reaction!

He turned to me and said, "There. You see, Ronald? The corneal reflex is one of the strongest reflexes in the body. Because she didn't move a muscle, or try to blink, when I tested it means that she is adequately anesthetized. Good job, my boy." As he left the room, he recommended that I should keep that technique in mind and use it frequently. It goes without saying that I never did that to any of my patients.

These days, protection of the anesthetized patient's eyes is a primary concern. After they're asleep, we routinely put some neutral ophthalmic ointment in each eye and then tape them lightly shut with hypoallergenic tape. Also, they are watched carefully in the recovery room so that in their half-awake state they don't inadvertently reach up to rub an eye and damage it.

I wonder how many patients over the years suffered corneal abrasions and/or permanent vision impairments at the hands of the old chief.

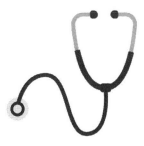

50. Two Car Crash Stories

Late one mid-winter evening, just as we finished up a case, the supervisor came into the OR to inform us that three people from a car accident on the highway had just arrived in the ER and that all three were badly hurt. News like this usually meant we'd be working all night so I quickly cleaned up my equipment and got everything ready for what was sure to be a few trauma cases.

When I got to the ER it was full of EMTs, paramedics, and nursing personnel hovering around the accident victims. It was a flurry of activity amid shrieks of pain! I asked the ER doctor which one was hurt the worst and would be going to surgery first, and he directed me to a young woman who had a smashed pelvis and whose right leg was twisted grotesquely almost 180 degrees backwards, with her knee bent the wrong way. Her face was covered with lacerations, probably from flying glass, and her mouth was a bloody mess with broken teeth, a bloody tongue, and ripped lips. There was a strong odor of alcohol coming from her. She was screaming in agony.

Fortunately, I had some fentanyl drawn up and with me so I introduced myself and gave her an IV dose of it which calmed her down immensely. She had a small IV in one arm, but I was pretty sure she'd need a lot of fluid, maybe even blood. I started a large bore IV in her other arm and as I did she said, "Could I ask you something? How soon before I can wear high heels again?" In my mind, I thought, *Seriously? With that horribly messed up leg? Probably never!* But between the alcohol and the fentanyl I'd given her, she drifted off before I had an answer.

We got her to surgery. Stabilizing all her fractures and sewing up all the lacerations on her face kept us there until almost dawn and the air ambulance from Minneapolis came for her later that day.

The other two crash victims, who had been in the same vehicle as the woman, were a couple of young fellows. One of them just had a broken and non-displaced fractured forearm, and the other had multiple facial lacerations, which they sewed up in the ER.

When we finally finished, I went out to the ER to see if there were any more trauma patients who might need surgery and the supervisor asked me how the woman's surgery went. After I explained her condition, I got the full story on the accident which the supervisor had heard from the sheriff. The two guys and the woman were very drunk and had just left a bar in town and gotten into a pickup truck heading home fifteen miles away on a busy highway. The woman was riding opposite the other two on the passenger side next to the door. The driver was so intoxicated that he evidently couldn't see the road well, and he was marking it by the oncoming headlights. He would drive right at them and swerve out of the way at the last minute. You can imagine what eventually happened. He didn't swerve in time and hit an oncoming car head-on at highway speed. The occupants of the car he hit were a father, mother, daughter, and three small grandchildren—all of whom were killed. The father just happened to be the principal of the high school where my wife taught English. They were riding in a small sedan—no match for a pickup truck.

The young woman sustained those horrible injuries because she had been riding with her right foot resting up on the dashboard and when the impact occurred, the dash caved in enough to twist her leg and drive the femur bone into her pelvis. Many months later, the doctor on call that night told me he'd heard that she was in Minneapolis and, after numerous surgeries, was still having trouble walking.

I wonder if she ever put on another pair of high heels...

During another middle-of-the-night call for a car crash on the highway, I was surprised to find a good friend of mine lying in the ER with a broken leg, broken arm, and facial lacerations from flying glass. He told me that he'd been driving back from Minneapolis and as he neared home, he noticed a set of oncoming headlights in the distance that appeared to be in his lane. As they got closer, there was no question they were in his lane. My friend pulled way over on the road, and the headlights did the same. Next, he pulled over on the shoulder of the highway and so did the headlights. Scared to death at that point, my friend drove down in the ditch and the oncoming headlights followed. As he was opening his car door to get away, the oncoming vehicle smashed into it. Fortunately, in the bumpy ditch it wasn't a high-speed impact.

He said that the other driver was really intoxicated and the highway patrol told him that the guy had been using oncoming headlights to mark the road. He wished he'd have pulled over and shut his lights off. The other driver wasn't hurt at all.

Luckily, my friend only had simple fractures and lacerations.

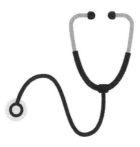

51. The Dentures

Before any surgery that involves general anesthesia, it's important to have all the patient's jewelry and nonpermanent teeth, dentures, bridges, etc., removed. In the '70s, all that was taken care of in the patient's room before bringing them to the OR. Jewelry was usually given to the person(s) there with the patient, and dentures were put into a cup and left in the patient's bathroom.

My first case one morning was a gall bladder removal (cholecystectomy) for a very pleasant, middle-aged lady. She was the wife of a prominent local businessman and was involved in many of the town's activities and charities. I had seen her the night before during my preop rounds and she mentioned that she had a full set of dentures but nobody had ever seen her without them, not even her husband—although he knew she had them. She asked if she really had to take them out. I told her about the kinds of airway issues that occurred while a patient was anesthetized and the possibility of complications if we left them in, but I consented to her taking them out in the OR immediately prior to being anesthetized.

We got her on the OR table and she dutifully took out her dentures, which the circulating nurse put in a labeled denture cup. I then proceeded with the induction of anesthesia. The case took an hour and was uneventful. The lady went to the recovery room and immediately upon awakening asked for her teeth. The nurse told her that they had sent them to her room, where she would be going shortly but the lady insisted they be returned to her immediately, so we decided to take her back to her room right then. After our patient left the recovery room and had been gone for a half hour, we got a call from the ward asking us to please send her dentures back to her. Our circulating nurse told them that she had put them in a denture cup, labeled it and sent it upstairs to her room with the orderly at the beginning of her surgery.

Now there was a big problem. They had scoured the room and couldn't find them. The orderly was questioned and insisted he put them in the bathroom on a shelf by the mirror. The housekeeper was also questioned but claimed never to have seen the cup. The laundry hadn't gone out for the day yet, and every bag in the linen room was opened and searched. Maintenance also opened every trash bag from that day, to no avail. The dentures had vanished and the poor woman was distraught! "It's bad enough that they got lost, but how many people here in the hospital now know that I have them?" she lamented. "It's bound to get into the community too. Until now, nobody except my husband and my dentist know it." She had a good point.

The lady refused to leave the hospital until she had a new set of dentures, so arrangements were hastily made. Her door was always closed with a big sign on it that read, "No entry, check with the nursing station." Her dentist visited her every day for a week. Finally, on her eighth postop day she got her new dentures and went home.

The hospital didn't charge her for anything and paid for all her dental work.

I saw her downtown a few weeks later. Although no mention was made of the denture debacle, she gave me a charming smile.

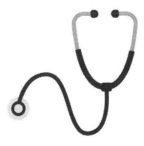

52. Holiday Prescription Refill

One morning in the late '80s, I was assigned to the pain patient room. These cases typically involved patients with intractable, chronic pain, often due to a post-spinal surgery in which hardware has been implanted.

The procedures were usually epidural steroid injections, accompanied by light sedation, plus a local anesthetic at the injection site. They didn't take long and everybody was an outpatient. Many of the patients had a long history of taking opioid medications which made their anesthetic requirements a bit challenging at times. Often, making sure their prescriptions were up-to-date was their main postop concern.

My third case that morning was a lady who fit the above description perfectly. As I wheeled her into the OR, right by her doctor standing at the scrub sink, she made me stop so she could ask him, "Dr. Johnson, don't forget to fill my pain medicine prescription and give me some extra pills, because a holiday's coming up. You know how I need them, and I don't want to run out."

He turned to her and in a droll voice said, "Let me see. I need to figure something out. Okay, I've got it. How would you like me to write you a prescription for all the pills you'll ever need for the whole rest of your life? It comes to about 250,000 pills. Got room in your medicine cabinet for that many?"

She thought for a moment and said, "No, I don't think so."

It took a great deal of self-control not to burst out laughing at that.

I wheeled her into the OR, got her sedated, and the case went well. Afterward, I told the doctor that he might have been more than just a little impertinent in his response to the patient. He told me that she calls his office weekly for prescription refills and is always running out.

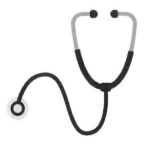

53. Resuscitation

A big April Fool's Day '50s party took place on the evening of April 1, 1977 at the Elks Club, BPOE 1052, in our little northern Minnesota town. Lots of people attended, including almost all the medical staff from the local clinic. It was a sorely needed gala to break up the monotony of a long, cold winter. The band played old music and everybody was having a good time.

About eight o'clock that night, as I was laughing and joking with some friends, I heard my wife scream out my name from across the crowded dance floor. I ran over to her and saw a very good friend of mine lying on the floor in what looked like a state of cardiac arrest. He had just finished a jitterbug dance with his wife. Immediately I felt for a carotid pulse and there was none. Fortunately, a lot of physicians were there too and we started CPR right away.

Those days, the standard of care was mouth-to-mouth resuscitation along with chest compressions. I performed the mouth-to-mouth and chest compressions were done by the doctors. My friend's family was there, and his son-in-law ran down to the bar and called 911. The police and ambulance crew arrived shortly and brought an AMBU bag and an oxygen tank which allowed me to do a better job of ventilating my friend. We got him on a stretcher and into the ambulance, still doing CPR, and the hospital wasn't far away so it didn't take long for us to get there. Once we were in the ER, a flurry of activity ensued to get my friend stabilized and moved to the ICU. He had a heart rhythm by then and was breathing on his own but was still only semi-conscious. His family members from the party had arrived and one by one they went in to see him.

Just before midnight he died. He was only fifty years old.

His daughter told me later that she was the last person to see him and when she spoke to him and squeezed his hand, he squeezed hers back.

My friend was very well known and loved by almost all the townsfolk. The only small consolation for me was that I was able to participate in keeping him alive long enough for his family to say goodbye.

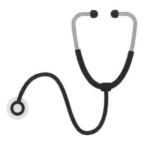

54. Unusual Delivery

One bitter-cold winter Wednesday morning, a call came into the OR that a car had just arrived in the ER with a woman in the back seat who was about to have a baby. I was working with our new lady gynecologist that day and, fortunately, we were between cases so she and I quickly rushed downstairs to the ER receiving entrance. There in the driveway was a dirty, beat-up, old four-door sedan that looked like it had been driven to the hospital through a hayfield. The driver, an unkempt young man, jumped out yelling, "Hurry, my wife's having a baby!"

We opened the back car door to the sound of a muffled groan, followed by the cry of a newborn. The doctor climbed into the car, exclaiming, "Oh, look at this beautiful little baby! What a good job you did, Mom!" The lady had pushed her baby out onto the filthy car seat which had pieces of straw lying here and there. I was with the ER nurse standing right by the open door and we noticed a hint of a barn odor coming out of the car. The doctor quickly clamped and cut the umbilical cord, then handed the baby boy out to the nurse who wrapped him in a couple of blankets and rushed him inside.

With the help of two orderlies, we got Mom onto an ER cart and took her inside too. The baby went upstairs to be cleaned up in a special section of the nursery, called the "suspect nursery," dedicated to babies born outside the hospital. Mom stayed in the ER until our doctor got the placenta delivered, then she went upstairs to be cleaned up too, since her appearance rivaled that of her husband's.

There are a lot of small rural towns in the large area surrounding Bemidji, some with a population only in the double digits. These folks had come from one of them and were part of a commune living out in the country.

Mother and baby did fine and were discharged after a few days. They had one unusual request, though: They wanted to take the baby's placenta home with them and eat it. According to what they told the nurses, it's a very healthy way to bond with your newborn.

There are even cookbooks for placentas.

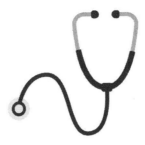

55. Two Blood Transfusion Stories

On a winter morning in 1969, while I was a senior student at one of the large Minneapolis hospitals, I got word that my cases that day were being moved and that an emergency traumatic amputation case was coming into my room right away. I asked my supervising CRNA what the injury was and she explained that while a man was loading groceries into the trunk of his car in a parking lot, another car pulled into the space behind him and because of ice on the pavement the second car couldn't stop and slid into him, crushing both his legs between the bumpers. She said the legs were beyond salvaging and needed to be amputated immediately to stop the bleeding. She also told me that the man's hemoglobin was dangerously low and that he would need a transfusion of at least two to three units of whole blood.

I got set up for the case right away and brought in a pressure transfuser. Next, the chief anesthesiologist called to tell me that the man had a religious belief that made him refuse blood and that he was yelling loudly about in the ER. When I asked him how we'd handle that, he said, "Nobody's going to die in my operating room because of that stupid belief. Now, Ronald, when he gets here and says it to you, humor him and let him think that you understand and will honor his wishes. I have a good friend who's a judge and he'll issue a court order declaring this guy incompetent to make that decision and, under the circumstances, we'll give him all the blood he needs and save his damn life. Do you understand me?" I told him I understood completely.

When the fellow came to the OR, he was an otherwise healthy man in his '60s, had been sedated, and was still mumbling about refusing blood from us. Fortunately, he never asked me directly about it so I never had to lie to him and

I just reassured him that he was in good hands. He had large bore IVs running in each arm and had received enough fluid in the ER to support his blood pressure, but he was white as a sheet. I'd never seen a hemoglobin value as low as his. We got him on the OR table and anesthetized quickly.

Both his legs still had tourniquets applied to them by the paramedics. They had been crunched right at the knees and were lying there askew, attached by only a few bits of muscle and skin. The injuries were filthy with debris from the road, pulverized knee joint material, and the heavy pants he'd been wearing that had been ground into them. As the circulating nurses were cleaning up his wounds and prepping him, the chief anesthesiologist came running in, exclaiming, "I've got it! My friend just signed the order, so we can proceed with whatever we have to do." Everybody cheered.

The case went well, and it took about four hours to amputate both legs above the knee, then irrigate, clean up, and close the incisions. By the end, I'd given him four units of whole blood and his color had returned and his vital signs were stable. I took him to the recovery room semi-conscious and gave the nurse report about the blood circumstance.

A week later, the chief told me that our former patient was mad as hell when he finally woke up and found out about the transfusions.

I never heard how that got resolved.

In the early '70s, techniques of ectopic pregnancy diagnosis were not as sophisticated as they are today. Ectopic pregnancy was always assumed as part of the differential diagnosis of any woman of childbearing age presenting with severe abdominal pain, and frequently the woman ended up having an exploratory laparotomy as the definitive means of diagnosis.

On a beautiful fall Saturday afternoon, I was called to the hospital for an emergency exploratory laparotomy on a twenty-six-year-old lady with abdominal pain. The ER nurse told me that the surgeon was pretty sure she had a ruptured ectopic pregnancy. When I saw her, she was basically healthy but in a great deal of discomfort and had a large bore IV in her arm. She was very pale, but her labs were all normal—except for a very low hemoglobin value coinciding with internal bleeding.

I asked the nurse if a blood type and crossmatch had been done. With her hemoglobin that low, she was sure to need a few units as soon as possible. To my surprise, the nurse told me that the testing had been done, but the patient was of a religious conviction that prevented her from ever having a blood transfusion, no matter the circumstance, and that she had signed, witnessed, and notarized papers to that effect. That was a shock to me, since she was sure to lose more blood before the internal bleeding was controlled.

I discussed my concerns with the surgeon, who told me, "Ron, we have to abide by her wishes and do the best we can. No judge in this town would go against her signed documents. It's in God's hands now." I asked him if a judge could declare her incompetent to make that decision, and he said, "Yes, they could, if she had made it in an altered state, such as she's in now, but she had these papers formally drawn up before all this happened, so we have to honor them."

We took her to the OR, and I anesthetized her using the rapid sequence induction technique because of her condition and questionable full stomach. It didn't take long for the surgeon to open her abdomen and find that it was full of dark, semi-clotted blood. When he'd sucked it all out it almost filled one two-liter suction bottle. He quickly found the ruptured fallopian tube and pregnancy, which was still bleeding, and ligated it. We were all concerned, since the lady was critically anemic preoperatively and with this added blood loss she would be lucky to survive without replacing it.

Her vital signs were very low at the end of the case due to her anemia. She had an adequate circulating volume but not enough red blood cells in it to sustain normal bodily functions for long. She was marginally awake at the end of the case and breathing on her own—but I left the endotracheal (breathing) tube in her with the idea that if she suffered a cardiac arrest we'd need it to ventilate her. Her postoperative lab work showed her hemoglobin was even lower than before. What a helpless feeling, to be dealing with such an easily treatable condition and be prevented from doing so.

I stayed at the hospital with the lady, consumed by an overwhelming feeling of foreboding. Early in the evening the lady's heartbeat became irregular, and she stopped breathing on her own. I was called to ventilate her and the surgeon was present as well. Nothing we did would straighten out her cardiac rhythm, and she was turning progressively cyanotic (dusky-blue skin color) from the lack of oxygen-carrying red blood cells. After an hour her heart finally flat lined, and we had to let her go.

It was awful. All the ICU nurses were in tears.

I never had to face another situation like that again in my career.

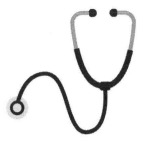

56. The Shoulder Block

In the late 1980s, regional anesthesia techniques weren't nearly as sophisticated as they are today. The anesthesia set-up for upper extremity surgery, from shoulder to hand, usually consisted of no more than a steel needle hooked to an extension set connected to a syringe full of local anesthetic. For shoulder surgery, the regional anesthetic of choice was—and still is—an interscalene brachial plexus nerve block. The brachial plexus is located on either side of a person's neck just above the collarbone (clavicle) and performing that type of block back then required a great deal of patient participation. When a needle was inserted into the neck, the patient had to tell the anesthesia practitioner what sensation they felt in their arm and where it was located. When the practitioner was satisfied that any sensation the patient reported corresponded to the approximate area of surgery, the local anesthetic mixture was injected which rendered the patient's shoulder and arm completely numb.

One morning I had a ninety-year-old man with significant medical issues on my schedule; he was in for repair of an upper arm (humerus) fracture. The attending anesthesiologist and I decided that he was too unhealthy to tolerate a full general anesthetic and that an interscalene block, plus light sedation, would be just perfect for him. At that time, all the nerve blocks we performed were done in the preop holding room. He was a very alert and well-oriented fellow and agreeable to the procedure after I explained everything to him. I put low flow nasal oxygen prongs on him and had an oxygen saturation monitor on his finger. I proceeded to find my landmarks on his neck, made a local anesthetic skin wheal there, and cautiously proceeded to insert the block needle.

He was tolerating everything well, and when he reported a shock all the way down his arm to his hand I knew I was in the right place. I aspirated (drew back on the syringe), injected a small precautionary test dose of the anesthetic mixture to make sure my patient had no untoward effects, and then waited a few minutes. When I asked him how his arm was feeling, I noticed that his voice was significantly weaker than it had been previously. As he continued to describe the sensation in his arm, he started to gasp. All of a sudden he couldn't talk at all and then stopped breathing completely. That gave me quite a scare!

Fortunately, the saturation monitor on his finger was beeping regularly, corresponding to his pulse, and his oxygen saturation was still above ninety. I called for the crash cart, which was brought over immediately by the nurse assisting me. Next, I put an endotracheal tube in his airway and began to ventilate him manually with an AMBU bag. I called for a ventilator, and with it came my attending anesthesiologist. The only explanation I could come up with for what happened was that my block needle had inadvertently slipped into the patient's cervical epidural space, and that's where the 3 ccs anesthetic test dose I'd given him had gone, effectively causing him to be paralyzed from the neck down until it wore off.

The man was still awake, so I gave him a small dose of tranquilizer and calmly explained the situation to him to allay his fears. The surgeon hadn't arrived yet and I was nervous about what his reaction would be when I told him what happened because he had a reputation of being somewhat irascible, and I hadn't worked with him before. I didn't have to wait long. When he arrived I took him aside to explain the situation. His first response was, "Damn, what a coincidence! I did the same thing to a young girl in my office the other day and had to do mouth-to-mouth on her 'til the paramedics arrived." Aside from being stunned, I was very relieved.

We kept the old man in the recovery room on the ventilator for an hour until the block wore off and he was fully awake, able to breathe normally again, and all his vital signs were stable.

Catastrophe averted. Needless to say, the case was canceled.

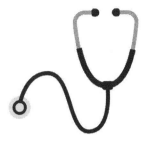

57. Bran Muffin

At our little hospital in the north country, all tissue specimens, except ones in immediate need of a frozen section, went into a labeled container in formalin and then into a basket to be sent to the lab at the end of the daily surgery schedule for our pathologist to examine. The pathologist would examine the specimen and dictate his report which would ultimately end up in the patient's chart. I knew the pathologist well since we'd both been at that hospital for years. He was well respected but a very serious—almost to the point of being humorless—soft-spoken fellow who smiled infrequently. A perfect foil for me.

One afternoon, as I was walking by the specimen basket in the OR, an idea for a small practical joke struck me. We still had a few muffins left in the break room from morning coffee, so I took one of them, put it in a specimen cup, labeled it "Please Identify," and placed it in with the other specimens for the lab then I finished my cases and left for the day.

The next morning as I walked by the OR supervisor's office she said, "Say, Ron, could I talk to you for a minute?" After I sat down, she began. "I got a call from the lab this morning, and the pathologist said he had received a very unusual specimen yesterday. So I asked him, 'Well, what does it look like?' He said, 'It looks to me like a bran muffin, and it was labeled 'Please Identify.' Immediately, I thought, I know exactly who did that. So I said to him, 'Oh, it must have been a joke.' He said, 'A *joke*! You know, once, about ten years ago, somebody played a joke on me!' I told him I'd ask the staff if any of them knew who did it." She and I had a good laugh over it. "Ron, you're a naughty boy," she told me.

These days you could never get away with something like that. You'd wind up in front of the administration immediately and probably be on probation for a long time—if they even let you keep working.

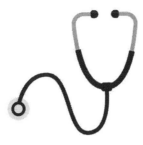

58. Bottled Water

One morning in 2010, as I was sitting at a desk in the preop department, I noticed a pleasant-looking middle-aged couple in the cubicle right across from me. The lady was the patient and lying comfortably on a surgery cart, with her husband sitting on a chair next to her reading the paper and holding a bottle of water. I was looking over the chart for my patient when suddenly I heard a loud crash, followed by a scream. The husband in the cubicle was now lying on the floor, twitching a little, and his wife was sitting up on the cart calling for help.

A bunch of us ran over to him and when we got there he was unconscious and had an extremely irregular pulse. We lifted him on to a cart, put oxygen on him, hooked him up to all the monitors, and saw that his EKG had multi-focal cardiac irregularities. We immediately called for a cardiologist and, after starting an IV, sent him to the emergency room just as he was starting to wake up. His wife's surgery was canceled and she went down to the ER to be with him. About an hour later, the cardiologist called to let us know that the man was fine, awake and doing well. When they did lab work on him, it revealed a significant electrolyte imbalance. His sodium level was extremely low (hyponatremia). It turns out that he was an avid runner and drank bottled water constantly to stay hydrated. His wife told them that he almost always had a bottle with him. Bottled water is usually devoid of any minerals or electrolytes, so what he in effect had been doing was diluting the electrolytes in his bloodstream and body to the extent that it caused a cardiac arrhythmia. In the ER he was treated with intravenous normal saline over several hours, until his blood work normalized.

A happy ending to what everyone thought was a heart attack in progress.

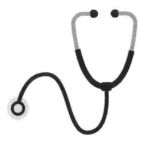

59. Craniotomy Insufflation

In the early 1970s, a well-respected neurosurgeon from Minneapolis liked to vacation in our little northern Minnesota town and he stayed at one of the area resorts where he enjoyed walleye fishing. One morning he woke up with chest pain and immediately came to the emergency room. It was determined that he'd had a small heart attack and was admitted to ICU, where he stayed for a few days until his cardiac tracing stabilized and he was then sent to a private room.

While there convalescing, he inquired about our capacity to perform emergency brain surgery (craniotomy) in the event a patient had a head injury causing intracranial bleeding. Our head trauma instruments at the time were old and sadly outdated. Upon learning this, the neurosurgeon decided he had to update our OR with all the latest craniotomy instruments. His cardiologist allowed him to go to the OR and help our supervisor order all the new equipment we'd need for an emergency craniotomy.

A few years after that neurosurgeon's visit, one Saturday morning in the summertime I was called to the hospital for what was suspected to be an intracranial (subdural) hematoma. Our patient was a young college student who had been hit in the head by a batted baseball. The old WWII-trained surgeon on the case assured me of the diagnosis and which side of the patient's head the bleeding was on.

When I saw the young man preoperatively, he was semiconscious and would only marginally respond to commands. According to his parents he was otherwise healthy, didn't take any medications, was physically fit and had only eaten a small breakfast of juice and toast a few hours before the injury. We brought him to the OR and I anesthetized him using the rapid sequence technique. Once he was asleep, I put a breathing tube in his airway (intubation), taped it securely into place on his upper lip, inserted an oral airway device in his mouth and turned on the anesthetic vapors. His head was shaved and prepped, then laid on a sterile cloth-wrapped foam donut, tilted thirty degrees to the side. He was lying supine on the OR table, sitting up at a ten-degree angle from the waist.

I was positioned away from the head of the table with all my equipment and sitting beside the patient, so that the surgeon had full access to the operative site. Because we didn't have the exotic anesthesia monitors in use today, it was considered important to keep an anesthetized craniotomy patient breathing spontaneously and assist their respirations as another method for assessment of anesthetic depth. Using all our new instruments, the surgeon made a scalp incision and proceeded to make an opening into the skull. Once it was open, he explored the area but couldn't find any evidence of bleeding at all.

"Well, I guess we'll just have to check the other side of his head," he announced, and with that he grabbed the patient's head and jerked it over thirty degrees the other way. Suddenly I lost my secure, pressurized airway. There was a big leak in the circuit, and I could smell anesthetic vapors escaping from under the drapes. I figured one of the breathing hoses had become disconnected, but when I checked under the drapes everything was connected perfectly. I also noticed that the endotracheal tube was hanging out of the patient's mouth about two inches further than where I had inserted it and the tape holding it in place was askew. The patient had a clear airway and was still breathing spontaneously because I could see the excursion of his chest and hear breath sounds in his lungs when I listened with a stethoscope. Nevertheless, he was obviously extubated since I heard breathing noises coming from his mouth.

Evidently, when the surgeon jerked the boy's head over to the side, that rapid motion had pulled my endotracheal tube back just far enough for the end of it to be out of his trachea and sitting in the back of his throat. After I crawled out from under the drapes, I announced my findings to everyone in the room. Needless to say, they were horrified! With his skull open and brain exposed it would have been risky and unsafe undraping him to facilitate a reintubation.

I remembered something from my school days: I had read about an old anesthetic technique called insufflation that had been in use years ago and I decided to give it a try. Nobody argued with me. Because the inhaled anesthetic gas mixture he was breathing was being diluted by room air, I turned the vapors way up to maintain an effective general anesthetic concentration. I monitored his vital signs and spontaneous breathing closely for about fifteen minutes and when I was satisfied that the patient's status remained stable and unchanged I told the surgeon to proceed. He opened the other side of our young man's head—and that's where the hematoma was. The surgeon irrigated and evacuated it, checked for bleeding, and closed up both sides of his skull and scalp.

It turned out to be an excellent anesthetic. I hadn't given our patient any narcotics, so when he breathed off the anesthetic gasses he woke up perfectly. He was oriented and, except for a headache, felt fine. We all breathed a sigh of relief. Of course, all the nurses thought I was a magician, which I allowed them to think.

When I called my old chief in Minneapolis and told him about the case, his only comment was "It's better to be lucky than good."

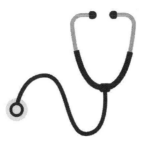

60. The Gas Sampling Line

Modern-day anesthesia machines are computer-driven, exotic pieces of equipment. Along with delivering exquisitely calibrated anesthetic gas mixtures, they have the ability to monitor almost every physical parameter of an anesthetized patient. Also, most routine monitoring is noninvasive and is transmitted to the computer screen for a comprehensive digital and graphic readout. This enables a CRNA to be immediately aware of the patient's status on a heartbeat-to-heartbeat continuum and at the end of the case the anesthesia record is available for printout as part of the patient's permanent record. As you might expect, there are a lot of tubes and wires connecting the patient to all these monitors.

One morning, a few years before I retired in 2018, my first patient of the day was an otherwise healthy middle-aged lady for laparoscopic cholecystectomy (gallbladder removal). This is an upper abdominal procedure which, because of positioning and intra-abdominal CO_2 insufflation, requires the patient to have an endotracheal tube inserted into their trachea during the procedure. After the induction of anesthesia, and insertion of an endotracheal tube, I connected the breathing circuit hoses from the anesthesia machine to the patient and turned on the ventilator, which I'd set to a normal respiratory pattern for her. In order to monitor concentrations of the inspired and expired anesthetic gas mixture, a very long gas sampling tube was connected from the computer module to the breathing circuit next to where the endotracheal tube was.

The circulating nurse was prepping the patient, the scrub technician was getting the instruments ready and I had all the drugs that I'd need for the case drawn up and on my anesthesia cart a few feet from where I was standing. As I turned to get one of the syringes, my right foot got tangled in the gas sampling line, which had fallen on the floor, and I started to stumble and fall forward. As I was going down, I saw all the equipment in front of me—my anesthesia cart and a three-foot-tall four-canister suction bottle stand—that I was going to hit. I glanced off the cart and landed on top of the suction apparatus with a loud crash before hitting the floor.

The circulator let out a scream and the scrub tech came running over to see what had happened. I didn't feel any excruciating pain, so I scrambled to get up and see how my patient was. To my horror, the jerk on the gas sampling line as I fell was enough to pull the breathing hoses loose from the anesthesia machine and completely extubate the lady. Now, her endotracheal tube was lying on the floor. With the circulator's help, we quickly changed out the breathing circuit on the machine and I opened up another sterile endotracheal tube and got her reintubated. This all happened in the space of about five minutes and the only injury I sustained was a small cut on my left hand. It could've been a lot worse.

When the surgeon walked into the room, all was well. Disaster averted.

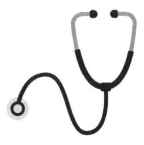

61. Tonsillectomy Experience

In 1970 I was a student CRNA rotating through five large Minneapolis hospitals for my clinical experience. One of them published a monthly newsletter for employees that was full of interesting articles relating to hospital events, and a section of it was devoted to interviews with patients about their recent hospital experience. My all-time favorite was the response a little four-year-old girl gave when she was asked what it was like when she had her tonsils out. She said, "Well, I really don't know, because when I went to the operating room they stuck me with a needle, and I disappeared."

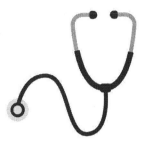

62. Frozen Buttocks

One bitter cold February Monday morning in 1970, when I was a student anesthetist at the county hospital in Minneapolis, my first case of the day was scheduled as a gluteal debridement on a sixty-seven-year-old man. This meant that the surgeon was going to remove dead tissue from the man's buttocks. I couldn't imagine what set of circumstances could possibly have led to a case like this.

When my patient arrived in the OR, I read the lengthy history on his chart. Two days before, he had been sitting outdoors on the steps of a downtown business's doorway drinking a bottle of wine and had eventually passed out, while sitting up and leaning against a wall. In his unconscious stupor, he had defecated and urinated on himself and the excrement had frozen his buttocks to the cement. A late-night passerby noticed him there barely breathing and had called the police. When emergency personnel arrived, they had to pour a few gallons of warm water underneath him to get his buttocks loose. He'd been in the hospital for a few days until it was quite obvious that the frozen areas were not going to survive and would have to be removed (debrided) and eventually skin-grafted. He was a pretty skinny fellow and malnourished-looking, but otherwise relatively healthy—with the exception of probably being a confirmed alcoholic. He needed to be watched closely for impending DTs.

I anesthetized him on the OR cart, secured his airway with an endotracheal tube, and we turned him over on his belly to the OR table. What an ugly sight his backside was! From the top of his buttocks to halfway down his thighs on either side, everything was dark purple and blackish with weeping dead skin peeling from it. The excrement had been cleaned off when he was admitted, and now all the tissues were sloughing and infected.

The surgeon said, "Well, we'll see what we can save, but he's so skinny it might go right to the bone, and it'll take a while for all this tissue to either live or die before we'll know what he's left with." The team picked off, cut away, and irrigated dead tissue from the affected area for a couple hours until it finally looked pinkish. At the end of the case, the whole area was a big, oozing, bloody mess. Large, absorbent dressings were applied, and it was quite apparent that we'd be seeing this fellow back in surgery many more times.

I stayed at the hospital until the end of March, and for a few weeks we saw this fellow every Monday, Wednesday, and Friday for more debridements. Finally, after two months, his doctors decided it was time to start skin-grafting the area. I had moved on to my next rotation by then, but classmates kept me informed of his progress. He was in the hospital another month getting skin grafts from many other areas of his body to his backside. One of my classmates told me that when that it was all finished, he saw the patient stand up—and the guy had absolutely no ass at all, just a flat area with a sphincter, which miraculously hadn't been damaged.

The only bright side to the whole ordeal was that with all the anesthetics and pain meds he'd received, he didn't suffer any withdrawals from alcohol.

I often wondered if he learned a lesson about drinking....

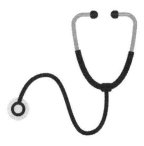

63. Sunflower Seeds

Bemidji is a beautiful northern Minnesota town surrounded by gorgeous big lakes and forests. In the summer, its population nearly doubles due to vacationers streaming in from all over the US—a fact that usually kept us busy at the hospital day and night all season long with various kinds of emergencies.

One weekday afternoon, I was notified that there would be an add-on bowel obstruction case coming to my room from the ER. I got my equipment all set up and went to see the patient. He was a healthy and embarrassed young man visiting from another state who admitted to having eaten a five-pound bag of sunflower seeds—along with the shells. He hadn't had a bowel movement in two days and he was bound up tight, despite having taken several different laxatives. An x-ray of his abdomen showed that he was plugged from his rectum up to his sigmoid colon. Rather than opening his belly, the surgeon decided he would try to remove the impaction from below.

After the patient was anesthetized and in a lithotomy position, the surgeon used his finger to do a digital rectal exam, during which he proclaimed, "I'll see what I can do, but there are ground-up sunflower shells as far as I can feel, and I have a long finger. I suspect he might have to come back at least once more to get thoroughly clean." He manually removed about half a surgical basin full of shells and did a saline irrigation up as far as he could. The fellow woke up fine and went back to his room on a clear liquid diet. We put him on the OR schedule again for the next day, assuming that if he couldn't pass the rest of the shells that evening, we'd clean him out then.

The next afternoon, we brought him back and repeated the procedure from the day before. This time the surgeon removed all the shells completely, another surgical basin full, and irrigated out the debris that was left. One of the nurses commented, "It's a good thing he didn't eat a ten-pound bag, or this would have been our case for the week."

I suspect he never ate sunflower seeds again.

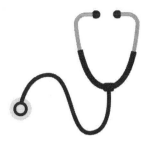

64. Pierre-Robin

Pierre-Robin syndrome/sequence is a congenital facial abnormality character-ized by an abnormally small mandible (lower jawbone), which causes a down-wardly displaced or retracted tongue and often causes breathing problems due to obstruction of the upper airway. It occurs in approximately one in ten thousand births and may also be associated with a cleft palate. Severe cases of Pierre-Robin are usually surgically corrected at a young age. Occasionally, in-dividuals with a mild case of this syndrome—without a cleft palate and severe mandibular deformity—are not corrected and live on to adulthood with it and, as you can imagine, are a challenge for anesthesia providers.

In 1970, when I was a student CRNA in Minneapolis, my first patient of the day for elective knee cartilage surgery appeared to have that problem. He was an otherwise healthy thirty-year-old man who had not had any pre-vious surgery. I'd read about Pierre-Robin syndrome but had never dealt with it clinically. In those days there was no preop holding area and patients came directly to surgery from the ward. The resident who had done his history and physical only made a brief mention of the airway findings in his notes, stating, "The patient appears to have a receding lower jaw." He actually had quite a significant overbite along with the receding lower jaw. I asked the fellow if he had any breathing problems and had him to stick out his tongue. He denied breathing issues, but when I examined his airway he couldn't open his mouth very wide and I could only see part of his tongue and couldn't see the back of his throat at all.

I was very uneasy about my patient's airway because I knew it would be next to impossible to get an endotracheal tube into his trachea or get a good mask fit to his face due to the overbite. Regional spinal anesthesia would've been the perfect choice. I called my attending anesthesiologist, who happened to be the chief of the department, and when he came into the room I explained the situation and all my concerns. He looked at the patient briefly and said, "Ronald, you just haven't done enough of these cases to know how to handle them properly."

With that, he picked up a full syringe of Pentothal and muscle relaxant and injected it into our patient's IV. The man immediately became unconscious and stopped breathing. I put the mask from my anesthesia machine on his face but could not get it to seal to be able to ventilate him. I put my laryngoscope in his mouth and couldn't even see the back of his tongue. Now the patient was turning slightly blue, so the chief held the mask forcefully on his face with both hands while I squeezed the breathing bag and it still leaked a lot.

I said, "I think this guy needs a trach right away." The orthopedic surgeon overheard me, rushed over to see what was happening, and immediately called for a general surgeon to come to our room and perform a tracheotomy. In no time, a surgeon from another OR came rushing in and the room filled with people hurrying around for instruments and prepping our patient's neck. The patient was purple by now and had an irregular pulse, but in less than five minutes the surgeon had his neck open and a tracheostomy tube in place so we could hook up the anesthesia machine's breathing hoses to it. Once we were able to ventilate him with 100 percent oxygen, his color came back to a nice normal pink and his pulse evened out to a nice regular rhythm. I shudder to think what his EKG tracing must have looked like during that ordeal.

He woke up about a half hour later and, after a lot of questions by a neurology resident, was deemed not to have had any brain damage. The case was canceled and we sent him to ICU for the night with a strict warning not to receive a general anesthetic until his airway was surgically corrected.

A month later I was called on to present a case to the quarterly combined surgery and anesthesia morbidity and mortality conference. Naturally, I presented this one but in generic form and without naming any of the participants. The group consensus during the conference was that extremely poor judgment had been used by giving this patient a general anesthetic. By then everyone knew who the anesthesia provider was who had caused the problem, but no one singled out the chief and he never said a word.

I often wonder what the outcome would've been if the man's attending surgeon hadn't overheard me say that he needed a tracheotomy.

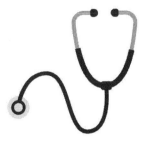

65. Queasy Husband

As previously mentioned, in the late '80s whenever I was called to obstetrics to perform a labor epidural I would always try to have the husband—or significant other—help me with positioning the patient. He would hold her steady in the event she had a contraction while I was working, and it would be a nice bonding experience for them. A labor and delivery nurse was usually on hand as well, keeping a close watch on the lady's monitors.

One afternoon I was called for a labor epidural on the wife of a very pleasant young couple having their first baby. They had been to prenatal classes, had seen all the videos and had dutifully practiced positioning and breathing and were quite well-informed about everything to do with the birthing process. It was busy in the department that day and as I was getting set up, the nurse asked me if she could step out for a little while to check on another patient. My patient was stable and very cooperative, so I told her to go ahead.

I had the lady sitting on the edge of the bed with her feet on a stool and her husband standing in front holding her in a fond embrace. We all enjoyed some nice, lighthearted conversation while I prepped her. I found my landmarks on her back, injected some local anesthetic and proceeded to slowly insert the epidural needle. While nearing the epidural space, I heard a loud crash in front of the lady. She started screaming her husband's name at the top of her lungs and moving forward away from me. Immediately I pulled the needle out of her back and grabbed her around the waist to keep her from falling off the bed. Her husband lay unconscious on the floor in front of us, having evidently fainted from being a part of this whole epidural process, and he had crashed into the bedside table on the way to the floor.

Now I started screaming, "*Hold still! Hold still! Nurse! Nurse, Help!*" Within a few seconds a couple of housekeepers, some aides and five nurses were in the room. I still had a firm hold on my patient because she was sobbing and shaking and precariously close to the edge of the bed. Thankfully, she wasn't obese or I might not have been able to keep her from falling. Her husband, still lying on the floor, had not stopped breathing and started to moan and wake up a bit. I told the folks in the room to get him over to the recliner chair and keep him flat, all the while trying to reassure the lady that they'd take good care of him and that he'd be fine and imploring her to please not move around. With help we got her lying down and as soon as her husband was in the recliner he woke up.

She was still sobbing and having frequent painful contractions, but when he told her he was all right and not to worry, she calmed down considerably. This all happened within the space of about fifteen minutes. She was progressing with her labor so this time, with her nurse's help, we got her sitting up and her epidural in place and functioning. In no time she was very comfortable, her husband was by her side in a chair, and they were smiling and deciding on names for their firstborn. He told me later that he'd always had a "thing" with needles and that when he saw the size of the epidural needle I was using he immediately started to feel queasy.

I wish he'd have told me that right away.

She went on to deliver a healthy seven-and-one-half-pound baby girl two hours later.

After that I never did another labor epidural without a dedicated nurse helper.

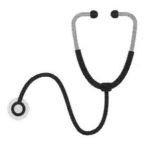

66. Tonsillectomy Tooth

In 1970, just after I graduated from anesthesia school and became a CRNA, I worked briefly at a large Minneapolis hospital. It had a rather large OR suite consisting of ten rooms, and ran a very busy daily surgery schedule.

My first case one morning was a tonsillectomy and adenoidectomy on a seven-year-old healthy little boy. The surgeon on the case was a young, board-certified ENT doctor whom I hadn't worked with much. In order to do this type of surgery, a special retractor is needed to hold the patient's mouth open so the surgeon has adequate exposure to his operative field. There are many types and sizes of mouth retractors, and whichever one is used is always a matter of the surgeon's preference.

After the child was anesthetized, intubated, prepped and draped, the surgeon opened his mouth and gently inserted the retractor. Its prongs were placed immediately behind the front teeth and worked with a ratchet mechanism to hold the retractor in place and the mouth open. The operation proceeded uneventfully but at the end of it, as the surgeon was removing the mouth retractor, it somehow snapped sideways hitting one of the child's front upper incisors and knocking it out. Luckily, the tooth fell outside of the mouth instead of down the throat. Everyone let out a gasp and the surgeon said, "Now I'll have some explaining to do to the parents."

I immediately called my attending anesthesiologist, who happened to be the chief of the department, to come and assess the situation. The surgeon was out of the room when he arrived, but after hearing what happened the chief was as angry as I'd ever seen him. The child woke up uneventfully and I explained everything to the surprised recovery room nurse. As I was walking back to my room to get ready for the next case, I passed by the main desk and heard the secretary tell the chief that the child's parents wanted to speak to him in the waiting room. He charged out of the department.

In about ten minutes he was back, fuming mad, and demanding to know where the ENT surgeon was who had done that tonsillectomy. He found out that the surgeon was in the locker room and quickly hustled over there, bursting through the door. The next thing I heard was a lot of screaming and yelling coming from the locker room, followed by sounds of shuffling—and possibly a body slamming against some lockers. After a few minutes the chief walked out, rubbing his hand and saying, "That son of a bitch found out the hard way about lying, and he'll never work here again. I should've knocked a few of his damn teeth out!"

It turned out that the surgeon told the parents that their child's tooth was knocked out by the anesthetist during placement of the endotracheal tube before surgery had even started. The surgeon stated that, though he was angry about it, he decided to proceed with the operation anyway. You can imagine what my irascible chief thought when he heard that. As he told me later, "When I confronted the asshole about his lie, he put his hand on my arm, and that was all it took. I punched him in the gut and slammed him into his locker and when he went down, I stepped over him and told him I was going to report him to administration and the state." Everybody within earshot clapped.

I was really proud of the chief because he, along with the chief CRNA, ran an excellent and no-nonsense, very busy department.

All my classmates loved the story too.

I never heard if the ENT doctor got reported to the state, but he never worked at that hospital again.

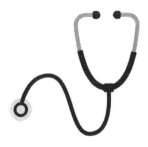

67. "Let Her Die"

One morning in 1973, while between cases, I was out on the ward to see my next patient who was already in the hospital waiting for his gallbladder surgery. As I passed one of the rooms, a nurse called out to me, "Ron, please come in here and have a look at this lady because as I was finishing her morning cares she passed out all of a sudden."

I hurried in there, noticed the lady was unconscious but breathing and immediately felt her pulse which was weak, thready, and very irregular. The nurse took her blood pressure at the same time; it was extremely low. I asked what the lady's diagnosis was, and the nurse replied, "Suspected MI [myocardial infarction—heart attack]." It seemed strange to me that a patient with that particular diagnosis wouldn't be in the ICU for close observation. I told her to call her doctor, have the EKG tech come up STAT and I got some oxygen on her since she was becoming cyanotic (a purplish-blue, dusky color to the skin from lack of oxygen and/or poor circulation).

The EKG tech arrived, hooked her up to his machine and within the first few seconds it was quite obvious to me that the lady was in the midst of a significant heart attack. Fortunately, her doctor was close by and arrived shortly. I told him what had happened and said that I wanted to intubate her and start CPR, because even though she had a pulse, she wasn't perfusing (her tissues). His response shocked me! He said, "No, this lady has had heart trouble for years, and even if we get her through this episode, she'll just be in with another one or die at home."

I told him that we could probably save her today and send her to Minneapolis for open heart surgery, which could give her many more years. His response was about as callous as I've ever heard: "No, she's been my patient for a long time, and I know she wouldn't want to go through all that. So, we'll just let her go peacefully today."

Her nurse and I just looked at each other, aghast! He made us stand there for the better part of a half hour, taking serial EKGs every few minutes, watching her turn blue and her heart gradually die. When she finally passed, he picked up all the serial EKG papers, put them in his pocket, and left the room, saying, "This will be very instructive in the coming years." The frustration and anger inside me was almost overwhelming. After he left, the patient's nurse and I had a long conversation about what a callous, awful doctor he was and how he needed to be reported to the authorities.

I didn't have much recourse after that experience. I reported it to the chief of the medical staff and hospital administrator, both of whom agreed with my assessment and said they'd look into it.

To my knowledge, nothing ever came of that incident, and the doctor in question went on to practice in town for many more years.

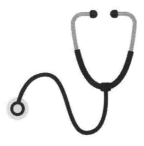

68. Bad Taste

In 1972 there weren't disposable gloves and hand-sanitizer dispensers everywhere in hospitals like there are now. The only gloves available then were sterile ones and once used they went to central supply for reprocessing and re-sterilization. Administering general anesthetics in those days was almost always done barehanded, with very few exceptions.

I was called to our little northern Minnesota hospital one late winter night for a bowel obstruction case on a seventy-year-old man. He was relatively healthy but had been experiencing abdominal pain for almost two days and he had been eating up until the present morning but now nothing he ate would stay down. His belly was quite distended and tender and he almost certainly had a stomach full of partially digested food. His lab work was all fairly normal, he had a large bore IV in his arm, had an adequate airway with no loose teeth, and was very uncomfortable.

The most important factor—all things being equal—in anesthetizing a patient under these circumstances is protection of the airway. With a stomach full of food and acid, there's always a possibility that some of that could come up and get into the patient's lungs (aspiration), causing all kinds of severe problems. The most critical time in administering an anesthetic under these circumstances is during the induction. There's a very brief period during which the patient goes from being awake with all his airway reflexes intact to asleep with no airway reflexes intact whatsoever. To facilitate making that period of time as brief and safe as possible, we employed a technique known then as a crash induction (now called rapid sequence induction). This is accomplished by sitting the patient up at a thirty-degree angle on the OR table, having the circulating nurse place pressure on the patient's neck just below their Adam's apple, and then rapidly injecting anesthetic drugs into the IV, followed by quickly inserting an endotracheal tube into their trachea the instant they lose consciousness. The cuff is then immediately inflated to seal off their airway, a technique which is still employed today.

After I had my patient safely anesthetized and our surgeon had his abdomen open, he felt the stomach and it was full so I inserted a nasogastric tube (NG tube) down his esophagus and into the stomach. This is usually accomplished by putting the lubricated NG tube into one of the patient's nostrils with one hand, and with the other one putting your index finger into the patient's mouth all the way to the back of their throat until you feel the NG tube coming down from the nose. Then you can guide the tube down the esophagus and into the stomach. I was able to suction out some stomach contents, but because of the partially digested food, the tube kept plugging up. Consequently, I had to keep removing it, irrigate the plugs out and reinsert it. This went on for the duration of the case until, at the end, his stomach was finally empty and the NG tube was draining properly.

The case lasted about three hours. By the time I had my patient awake and over to ICU and had cleaned up all the anesthesia equipment, it was 4 a.m. and I was dead-tired. I dragged myself out to the car and headed home. I lived twelve miles from town out in the country, and about halfway home I noticed a piece of the snack I'd eaten before the case stuck in one of my back teeth. I reached back there with my finger to get it out and immediately noticed a funny taste in my mouth. There was no mistaking that taste—it was stomach acid! In my dead-tired state after the long case, I'd forgotten to wash my hands after they'd been in the patient's mouth.

Waves of nausea swept over me, and I had to pull over on the shoulder of the road and throw up in the ditch. Between vomiting sessions, I'd take a handful of snow to rinse my mouth out and then wretch some more. When I finally got home, I was wide awake and spent the better part of a half hour brushing my teeth and gargling with mouthwash.

For a long time afterward, whenever I thought about it, I almost had that same taste in my mouth.

And I never forgot to wash my hands again.

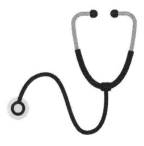

69. The Gold Grill

A laryngeal mask airway (LMA) is an elliptical-shaped device made of soft silicone with a hole in the middle of it that is attached to a tube that then connects to the breathing circuit of an anesthesia machine. It is designed to sit in an area of the throat (supraglottic) where the esophagus is, effectively sealing it off so that ventilation can take place in the trachea via the hole in the LMA. This airway device is used to maintain control of a patient's airway when the anesthesia requirements of a particular case don't require using an endotracheal tube.

These days, it's not uncommon to see a person with bright-gold upper front teeth. They can be caps or, in many cases, a "grill" that fits over the teeth like a mouth guard, and can be removed.

One morning, one of my first cases—for a small inguinal hernia repair—was a young fellow with a bright-gold grill over six of his upper front teeth. It had star-shaped openings in it so you could see his teeth through them. As I examined his airway, I asked him if he could take the grill out to ensure nothing would happen to it. He told me that a long time ago, right after it was made, he took it out once. For the last few years, however, he'd just left it in the entire time and now it was stuck and he couldn't get it out. He also told me the grill cost him several thousand dollars. The teeth that were showing through the star openings in the grill were none too healthy-looking either; they were all dark brown and probably in an advanced state of decay.

I asked him if those teeth hurt at all, and he said that they had a few years ago, but after a while the pain finally stopped. I put on a glove and very gently grasped them to see if they were loose. I thought I detected slight movement but wasn't positive. I told the young man about a special airway device we used (LMA) to keep him breathing while he was asleep and that I would be extremely careful of his front teeth and grill, but I was worried about what shape his teeth were in. I warned him that they might be so bad they could possibly break off. His only reply was, "Oh, okay. Whatever."

I anesthetized him on the OR table and very carefully opened his mouth to slide a well-lubricated LMA in. I had purposely used a slightly smaller LMA than usual because of the status of his teeth, and all went well. Next, I called everyone in the room over to have a look at his grill in the event something happened to it as he was waking up, because I wanted them all to know the situation.

The short case was uneventful, and at the end of it I had the patient lightly anesthetized and breathing spontaneously. I wanted to get that LMA out of him before he had a complete return of all his airway reflexes so he wouldn't bite down on it. I got it done, but a second afterward he let out a massive sneeze, stuck out his tongue, and out came the grill—rotten teeth and all. Fortunately, everything fell on the gown across his chest instead of down his throat. I grabbed the grill and had the circulator put it in a labeled specimen cup to go with him. We took him to the recovery room, and the first thing he did when fully awake was yell out with a lisp, "Whereth my grill?" I think he was more worried about the gold than his teeth. Once he saw it in the specimen cup he calmed down.

I think there's a lesson in here somewhere...

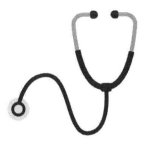

70. Rock Star

One morning in 2003 I was working with a talented and very congenial plastic surgeon friend of mine. He was a music lover and had quite a wide assortment of tunes on his iPhone. He would always ask the personnel in his room what they would like to hear in the background during surgery which made for a very pleasant working environment in his OR.

The case was progressing well that morning. After about two hours into it, one of my partners arrived to give me a break. I left and as I was sitting in the lounge, I received a text from my wife letting me know that a famous rock musician had just died. I wasn't familiar with the singer, but I knew my plastic surgeon friend would recognize the name. I headed back to my case, and upon entering the room announced to everyone that I'd just received a text from my wife telling me that Robert Plant had died. My surgeon friend snapped to attention with a horrified look on his face. "*What? Oh, no!*" He cried, and put his instruments down for a moment, looking almost stricken. The rest of the case went well, but after that news my friend became relatively quiet and contemplative. The surgery ended on that note and I took my patient to the recovery room.

When I got home that night and told my wife how upset my friend was after hearing the news, she said, "Oh, my god! It was Robert Palmer, not Robert Plant. Did you really tell him that?" I said yes, but I sure hope he found out the truth when he got home.

The next day we weren't working together but I when saw my friend in the staff lounge he said to me, "You know, Ron, after you told me that about Robert

Plant, I was really upset all day—until I got home and found out it was actually Robert Palmer who died."

That pretty much ended any credibility I might've had in the department about music and nobody asked me what I wanted to listen to during a case ever again.

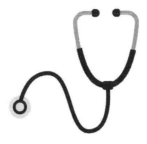

71. Linen Cart

In the late '60s I worked as a student CRNA in a large Minneapolis hospital that had a busy daily surgery schedule and performed all types of operations, except open heart procedures. The OR was laid out in an L shape, with five surgeries and associated supply rooms on each arm.

One weekday morning, as I was leaving the recovery room to get ready for my next case, I heard an overhead page in the OR for a certain surgeon to come to his room STAT because of an emergency with his patient during the induction of anesthesia. Immediately a surgeon burst out of the lounge and passed by on my right, running down the hall. The OR he was headed toward was around the corner and almost at the end of the hall, so he was really moving fast. It was mid-morning, and the housekeeping staff was in the OR resupplying our linen, taking one big linen cart out and replacing it with a fully stocked one.

About the time the running surgeon had almost reached the corner of the OR to make his turn, a housekeeper from one of the linen rooms was pushing her empty linen cart out the door and into the hallway. The timing couldn't have been more perfect, and the surgeon ran into that huge cart with a booming crash—which was heard throughout the whole department—and then fell limp to the floor. A bunch of us rushed over to see how he was. Fortunately, we found him dazed but awake and with a gash in his forehead and a sore shoulder and knee. The linen cart was bent and wedged into the doorway, causing the frightened housekeeping lady in the room behind it to yell for help, unaware of what had happened.

A couple of orderlies got the surgeon on a cart and took him to the recovery room, and the rest of us managed to unseat the linen cart to let the scared housekeeper out. She was very upset, having assumed she'd caused the whole disaster, but finally calmed down after accepting that it had been unavoidable. Meanwhile, the patient in crisis had been stabilized by anesthesia personnel, and a partner of the injured surgeon did the case so he could get his head sewed up and x-rayed.

It was the topic of conversation in our OR for a long time.

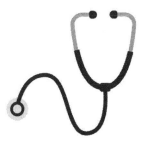

72. Grouse Hunter

Fall season always brought a lot of hunters to Bemidji. The huge area of woods surrounding our little town offered prime hunting grounds for grouse and deer, and it wasn't unusual to occasionally hear gunshots in the distance. Hunting season also brought us a lot of emergency cases from gunshot wounds, falling-out-of-tree fractures, game-cleaning knife injuries, and heart attacks from out-of-shape hunters dragging deer carcasses out of the woods.

One October morning I got a call from the emergency room that a gunshot victim was coming in who had been hit by a shotgun blast at close range. It was hard to imagine anybody surviving that, but I hurried to the hospital to set up my room and prepare for something terrible. Horrible worst-case scenarios were already being conjured up in my mind.

I got to the ER just as they were bringing in a scared young boy covered with blood from head to waist. He was in his hunting clothes; his jacket was torn to shreds around his left shoulder, and the left side of his face was peppered with red marks that had little black spots in the middle. The worst area was his left neck and, after we removed the heavy dressings the ambulance attendants had applied, it showed a gaping, bloody wound in it about the size of a grapefruit from his jawbone to the top of his shoulder. It wasn't bleeding much—just oozing. I was amazed that I didn't see blood pumping out of it from one of the big vessels there. The kid was awake and alert but scared to death.

Fortunately, he wasn't having any respiratory distress (dyspnea). He tried to talk and made sounds but couldn't phonate well enough to articulate words. I told him not to try to talk but to just lie quietly and breathe easy. His vital signs were stable, and we immediately put oxygen on him, got him undressed and inserted a large bore IV into his arm. I was very concerned about his airway because of swelling, displacement from the blast and bleeding. I told the attending surgeon that I needed to see if I could get him intubated immediately, before anything else, and after that he should have a tracheostomy tube in place until everything was healed.

His father and brother were present at the time of the accident and had accompanied the boy to the hospital. The father told me that they were from Minneapolis and were up in our area grouse hunting. They were walking in the woods abreast, about thirty feet apart, with our young patient in the middle. A bird flew up between the patient and his brother and the brother swung around to shoot, not paying attention to the fact that his brother was in the line of fire, and the blast hit his brother in the neck. Probably the only thing that saved the young kid from a much worse fate was the fact that there was a rather dense bramble bush half way between the shooter and our patient that took the bulk of the shot, and they were using very small pellets (#8 shot) in their 20-gauge shotgun shells.

I had the young fellow open his mouth and I could see the back of his tongue and throat. He could take a slow, deep breath and blow it out forcefully, which was a good sign, and I didn't hear any wheezing or chest congestion. I explained my concerns about his airway to him and his father, and I now felt that time was of the essence because of swelling and that he needed to be intubated immediately, followed by a tracheostomy. They were so frightened that they agreed to everything right away. I was concerned about him having a full stomach, but his dad said he hadn't eaten for five hours before the accident because they were up early hunting.

I had all my airway equipment and the drugs I'd need with me, so I explained to the young fellow what I was going to do and what would happen after he had a tracheostomy. The poor kid was so scared that tears were streaming out of his eyes. Next, I propped him up at a thirty-degree angle on the ER cart and had a Yankauer oral suction device ready. The ER nurse put a glove on and gently placed pressure on his Adam's apple (cricoid pressure), away from the blast injury. I gave him a small dose of sodium pentothal, followed by rapid acting muscle relaxant and carefully inserted my laryngoscope blade into his mouth.

As the blade approached the base of his tongue, I could see his vocal cords and the open airway between them, but the structures were deviated way over to the right of midline, and there was a lot of soft tissue swelling and I could see some small shotgun shell pellets just under the surface of his mucous membranes. I quickly inserted an endotracheal tube and inflated the cuff to seal his airway off. What a relief to have that secured. As the sodium pentothal and muscle relaxant wore off, the young fellow started to wake up and become agitated by the irritation of that tube in his throat so I gave him a dose of Innovar, which made him very relaxed and comfortable.

We took the young man to the OR and, after I anesthetized him, we explored, irrigated, and cleaned up his gaping neck wound. He had to be one of the luckiest people on earth that day because his injury was all soft tissue. If he had sustained a tear in his carotid artery, he'd never have made it out of the woods alive.

We brought him to the operating room a couple days later for a second look at his neck and ultimately we sent him back to Minneapolis in the air ambulance for further surgery and the possible skin-grafting he'd need and to close the blast wound and to remove his tracheostomy.

I wonder if he ever went grouse hunting again.

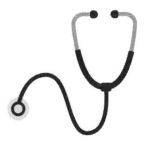

73. Unusual C-Section

As I mentioned previously, all anesthesia for cesarean section operations were done with general anesthesia in our little hospital in the early '70s. The patient was prepped and draped while awake on the operating table. When that was finished, I'd give the lady an induction dose of sodium pentothal and muscle relaxant and the minute she went to sleep, I'd give our gynecologist the okay to make his incision while I intubated the patient. This worked well and the surgeon would usually have the baby out in just a few minutes.

My first case one morning in 1973 was a C-section on a very pleasant, healthy, thirty-year-old lady and it was her first child. She needed this operation because the baby was full-term and lying transverse in the uterus instead of head-down. She was so happy that she was about to give birth, and all the OR staff was happy for her.

After she was anesthetized, the surgeon made his incision and had the baby out in just a few minutes. Horror of horrors, the newborn was a little girl but anencephalic—a rare disorder that occurs in about 1 in every 10,000 babies born and is characterized by a complete absence of a major portion of the brain, skull, and scalp. It occurs during embryonic development and these babies can be stillborn or live for a few minutes or a few hours after birth. The surgeon handed the baby off to the circulating nurse, who placed her in a bassinet right next to me.

I had never seen anything like that and was shocked by her appearance: just two big eyes and no head behind them. The baby made some gurgling sounds for a few minutes and then expired. It had a terrible effect on everybody in the OR and many of the nurses got pretty emotional. After the gynecologist was finished, he went over to his portfolio, pulled out the x-ray of our patient's abdomen and put it on the view box. The baby could quite plainly be seen lying transverse in the uterus. Also quite obvious was the fact that there was no cranium at the top end of the baby's spine. He remarked, "How on earth did we miss this?"

We all knew it would be a very difficult time in the recovery room after this nice lady was awake so the bassinet, with the newborn still inside and wrapped up, was taken to an empty patient room so the father and grandparents could all be there alone with the doctor to discuss everything. I gave her a dose of narcotic and tranquilizer so that when she woke up she wouldn't have much incisional pain and, hopefully, would be calm enough to deal with these awful circumstances. Before I woke her up, I decided that she should also go to a private room out on the ward with a recovery room nurse instead of in the OR where other patients were. They put her in the room with her baby so the family could all be together.

The first questions she asked as she was waking up and we were wheeling her out to her room were, "How's my baby? Is it a boy or a girl?" I just told her, "Dad's with the baby, and I'll let him tell you everything."

I still think about that case and I've never seen another one like it in my career.

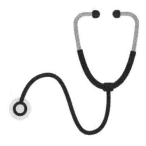

74. The Bezoar

In the mid-1970s one of my morning cases was on a ten-year-old girl scheduled as a gastric exploration for a foreign body. The diagnosis was gastric outlet obstruction. The surgeon showed me her x-ray, which revealed a mass in her stomach about the size of a golf ball. He was pretty sure it was a bezoar but wasn't positive what it was from. A bezoar is a solid mass of indigestible material that accumulates in the digestive tract or stomach that can possibly cause a blockage. It can develop from many different sources.

Our patient was a very pleasant child and let me start her IV without any problems. After I had her anesthetized and intubated, the surgeon made the abdominal incision. When we opened her stomach, it was just as he had suspected: a bezoar and it was made up of hair (called a trichobezoar) that matched the color of our patient's hair exactly and was almost perfectly round. He removed it and irrigated her stomach. I put down a nasogastric tube, and he closed her up.

It turns out, according to her parents, the little girl had long hair and a habit of chewing on it. Obviously, she'd swallowed a certain amount over the years until it finally became a problem. She woke up in the recovery room afterward and was fine.

I've seen many bizarre objects in different bodily orifices over the years. Plastic utensils and razor blades in the stomach, pencils in the urethra, beans stuck in the nose and ears, and pennies in the trachea, but never a hair bezoar in the stomach. I even had a patient on several occasions that we called "battery boy" who would swallow five or six double-A batteries and then present himself, smiling, to the ER. We'd dutifully bring him to the endoscopy unit, put him to sleep, and fish them out. After about three occurrences of this kind of behavior, we never saw him again.

Maybe he electrocuted himself...

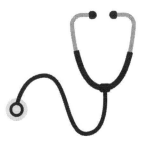

75. Perforated Bowel

One mid-morning in 1988, I was notified that an emergency perforated and septic bowel case was coming into my room right away. These kinds of patients can be extremely sick depending on how long their bowel has been perforated before they sought treatment. I quickly got all my drugs and equipment set up and asked the surgeon what our patient was like. The surgeon described him as a relatively healthy, middle-aged and moderately obese man who had what looked like a foreign body high enough up his rectum to perforate the sigmoid colon. The surgeon assumed it must have been there for a while, because he was a "sick cookie."

Our patient came straight to my room from the ER with a large bore IV in each arm and was moaning loudly. I gave him a dose of fentanyl to ease his pain, and we got him on the OR table quickly. Because of the bowel involvement, and possible full stomach, I anesthetized him using the rapid sequence induction technique. It didn't take long for our surgeon and his assistant to open the patient's abdomen and find his bowel perforation. There was a tear in his sigmoid colon that had one end of a large dildo sticking out of it. The surgeon pulled it out and handed it to his assistant, who inadvertently pushed a button on it, and it began to vibrate. I couldn't help but ask if the patient was going to get it back. "No way," said the surgeon.

After the surgery was finished, we brought our patient to the recovery room. He was sleepy from the narcotics I'd given him during the procedure but was just starting to wake up. I gave the nurse report and, as I was finishing my charting, our patient woke up fully screaming the filthiest language imaginable, calling the nurses terribly profane names, ordering them to get their hands "the f*ck off me," and using every possible foul epithet you can think of. I quickly ran to my room and got some more narcotics to sedate him, which did the trick and put him into a very comfortable half-awake and quiet state. Fortunately, he didn't stay long in the recovery room.

As I turned in my charting and billing papers from the case, I happened to notice on one of his admitting forms that he was a minister.

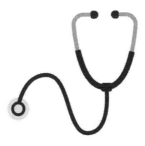

76. Squirt in the Face

Most cesarean sections these days are done using a regional anesthesia technique. The regional anesthetic of choice is frequently an epidural with an indwelling catheter, so that after surgery it can be left in place and attached to a pump that meters in continuous-flow local anesthetic to keep the patient happy and without incisional discomfort for a few days.

One morning in the early 1990s, my first case of the day was a cesarean section on a healthy young woman who was at full-term with her first pregnancy. These cases were all done in the obstetrics department located one floor below surgery. I went down to see the patient well ahead of time to establish a rapport with her and her husband and get her epidural in place in the birthing room so as to save time in the OR. Our surgeon that day was a lady obstetrician whom I knew quite well and had worked with many times. She was to be assisted by her male partner, also an obstetrician.

I put the lady's epidural in without a problem while her husband held her sitting up in a fond embrace. They were such a pleasant couple and just as I was finishing up, her surgeon came in for any last-minute questions. We laughed and joked for a bit and then off we all went to the OB surgery suite.

My patient was already a little numb in all the right places from the test dose of anesthetic I'd given her in the birthing room, and once we had her on the OR table, I gave her a full dose of it through the epidural catheter which made her completely numb from her rib cage to her toes. The circulating nurse was washing her belly while I hooked up all my monitors. Once we had her prepped and draped, we brought her husband in dressed in surgical garb to sit in a chair next to us at the head of the table. They were so happy while bantering with the obstetrician and me about names for the baby and how the whole family would be so excited to see their first grandchild.

The surgeon and her partner made an incision and had the baby out in about five minutes. A beautiful baby girl! She showed the little crying cutie pie to her parents and then handed her off to a waiting neonatologist for examination and determination of her APGAR score. The little girl was adjudged to be very healthy, so the neonatologist wrapped her up and brought her over to her parents. I loosened Mom's non-IV arm so she and Dad could hold her baby. It was truly a Hallmark moment. Then Dad got to hold his little girl and follow the neonatologist out to the nursery with her.

I lightly sedated the lady while the doctors started her abdominal closure. The two partners were having a conversation and as I listened, it became quite obvious that it wasn't particularly friendly. The lady surgeon was berating her partner over something to do with their office practice and every time he attempted to say something she spoke over him, using some pretty harsh language. Finally, the uterus was closed and her partner wasn't needed anymore for the abdominal closure, so he broke scrub and left the table.

As he walked by me to leave the room, I said to him, "You'll get your reward in Heaven."

The lady surgeon overheard and said to me, "What did you just say to him?" I responded, "Oh, nothing."

She replied with, "I said, 'What *in the hell* did you just say to him?'"

So, I told her.

"Damn you," she snapped, then picked up a 50 cc syringe, filled it up with the bloody saline that she'd just irrigated the patient's abdomen with, reached over the drapes and squirted the whole thing into my face at almost point-blank range. Talk about shocked! It's fortunate that I had glasses and a mask on. It splashed off me and down onto my patient's face, which woke her immediately. She asked me what happened an as I wiped her face, I had to lie and tell her it was just some sterile saline, and I quickly gave her more sedation.

I was wet from my face down my chest and abdomen with that bloody mixture; some of it even drizzled into my underpants. I didn't dare say anything because of the volatile state the surgeon was in and I was afraid of what might be next. The nurses in the room were as shocked as I was and just stared at me and the doctor, not daring to speak. I picked up a towel, wiped my glasses and face and the circulating nurse got me a new mask and cap.

Finally, the case was over, and not a word was spoken as the surgeon left the room. After she was gone, though, we said plenty—until the patient woke up. We took her back to her room where Dad and baby were waiting. Lots of laughter and congratulating ensued.

I left the OB department and headed back to the OR. As I entered the surgery suite and walked by the supervisor's office she saw me and asked, "What on earth happened to you?" I told her that I had accidentally been splashed with the liquid and kept walking to go change my scrub suit. A little later, when I came out of the dressing room, after cleaning up and changing scrubs, she saw me and told me that she had called OB to find out exactly what happened and they'd given her all the details of the incident. She went on to say that she was reporting it to administration. That was the last I heard of it because neither I nor the supervisor discussed it with anybody, not even the chief of my anesthesia group.

I didn't work with that lady doctor again until months later, when a morning assignment happened to be a gynecological case with her in the OR. I had some slight uneasiness about doing a case with the woman because I wasn't sure what to expect since I'd heard that after our incident in OB, administration demanded she go to anger management or lose her hospital privileges. She walked into the room before she'd scrubbed for the case, saw me and said loudly enough for everybody to hear: "Our office got a lunch yesterday from the cafe your wife owns, and nobody spit in mine, so I ate it."

That made me red-hot mad! I immediately called for my attending to come relieve me for a minute and then said to her, "Get your ass out in the hall! I have some things to say to you." My attending came right in to relieve me, and when I confronted her in the hallway, I said, "Listen, dammit. I know exactly what you had to go through because of that stupid squirt in the face you gave me in OB and I want you to know that I didn't say anything to anybody about it. When I came back to the OR that day sopping wet, the supervisor saw me and called OB and found out everything. You got exactly what you deserved and if you so much as look sideways at me or give me an ounce of trouble ever again, I'll go straight to the law and file an assault charge against you." She stared at me, wide-eyed, but never uttered a peep. Our case together that day went very well.

After that exchange, we worked together for quite a few more years and not a word was ever mentioned about that distasteful episode and our relationship even became quite congenial.

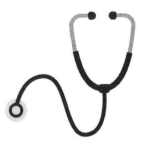

77. The ACL Repair

Our anesthesia group provided services to three surgicenters in addition to the hospital in St. Petersburg, Florida. Whenever I was assigned to one that did predominately orthopedic surgery, I usually worked with two extremely talented orthopedic surgeons and it was always a busy day.

Late one afternoon, we were finally on our last case: an anterior cruciate ligament (ACL) repair. Our patient was a large, burly, middle-aged man with a short bull neck and large mouth and tongue. He had an automatic implantable cardiac defibrillator (AICD) in his upper chest that was turned off and, according to the cardiologist's report on his chart, was scheduled for removal at a later date. He was from Haiti and had a significant French accent but seemed to understand all my questions during our preop interview. I examined his airway and thought it might be a bit of a challenge getting an endotracheal tube into his trachea, so I discussed the issue with my attending anesthesiologist. We ultimately decided that we could do it.

After our patient was on the OR table, I had him breathe 100 percent oxygen for a couple minutes before I gave him an induction dose of Propofol and muscle relaxant. After he went to sleep, I put the laryngoscope blade in his mouth but had trouble seeing landmarks in his throat because of his large tongue flopping in the way. After a few unsuccessful attempts, I finally saw the tip of his epiglottis and was able to slip an endotracheal tube underneath it and drop it into the trachea (a combination of luck, skill, and experience). Next, I connected the endotracheal tube to the breathing circuit on my anesthesia machine and gave him a few deep breaths of oxygen while my attending listened to his chest with a stethoscope to make sure both lungs were being equally well-ventilated, which they were.

I noticed immediately, however, that his oxygen saturation, which had been running at 100 percent, began to drop into the low 90s. I listened to his lungs again; both were still well-ventilated, so I called for my attending anesthesiologist to help me figure out what was happening. When he arrived and listened to our patient's breath sounds, he was as perplexed as I was. We changed all the oxygen saturation probes and wires, thinking it might have been just a connection problem, to no avail. The low oxygen saturation persisted, and because of this issue, the patient was still only being ventilated with 100 percent oxygen—I hadn't turned on any of the anesthetic gas vapors. This also meant that he might wake up with everything going on and an endotracheal tube in place, which would not be good.

I had to continually administer incremental doses of Propofol to keep him asleep. Fortunately, with high flows of pure oxygen, I could keep his saturation between the high 80s and low 90s. My attending anesthesiologist and I could not figure out exactly what was going on with our patient. The only explanation we came up with was that it must have something to do with the reason he had that AICD implanted in the past. Though he was receiving adequate oxygen ventilation it wasn't perfusing his tissues now that he was asleep.

Because our patient was in such a precarious situation, I mentioned to my attending that we needed to cancel the case because if we proceeded under these circumstances we'd probably have a life-threatening crisis in the middle of it, and with his knee opened surgically it could become a worst-case scenario. He agreed and explained the situation to the orthopedic surgeon, who felt the same way and said to me, "Ron, I don't need much more of an explanation than you telling me the case needs to be canceled because of concern for my patient's well-being." That was what we needed to hear, and immediately we had our circulator call for an ambulance to take our patient to St. Anthony's hospital in downtown St. Petersburg, Florida.

Twenty minutes later, the ambulance crew arrived with two paramedics and two EMTs. They were pretty wide-eyed, since none of them had ever been in an operating room, let alone a situation like this. I told them, "This patient is very delicately balanced right now. He's anesthetized at the moment, and we are having trouble keeping his oxygen saturation normal. It's been running in the high 80s to low 90s, and we're hyperventilating him with 100 percent oxygen. Also, he's not receiving any anesthetic gasses, so unless I give him incremental doses of Propofol, he'll wake up. Fortunately, his vital signs are relatively stable to a little on the high side. One of you has to be focused and dedicated to his ventilation with 100 percent oxygen, and one of you has to be diligent in watching all his vital signs. You can't be distracted for a second, and he needs to get to St. Anthony's as fast as he can to be in ICU and evaluated by a pulmonologist. Get everything ready, do what you have to do and come get him. One more thing: When I stop giving him Propofol, he'll start waking up fairly rapidly in the ambulance. I'll give him a good-sized dose of Versed and muscle relaxant now, so when that happens it'll dull the experience for him and maybe give him amnesia of it down the road."

With that, they sprang into action and had our patient on their stretcher and into the ambulance in no time. As soon as they left I called my chief anesthesiologist, Dwight Valentine, at St. Anthony's and explained the situation asking him to meet the ambulance when they arrived there.

Epilogue:

Our patient arrived safely at St. Anthony's and was immediately put into ICU on the ventilator. A pulmonologist saw him, but because I had been working at surgicenters and never got to ICU, to this day I'm not sure what his diagnosis was determined to be. I heard that he was there and on the ventilator for three days and eventually he was discharged.

Disaster averted!

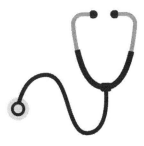

78. Omphalocele

An omphalocele is a relatively rare birth defect in which the infant's intestines and/or other abdominal organs are outside of the body because of a hole in the belly button (navel) area. The intestines are only covered by a thin membrane and can be easily seen. Survival rate is over 90 percent if that's the only problem.

Very early one Sunday morning, I received a call to come to the hospital right away for a baby in the nursery having respiratory distress because of a birth defect. I got there in about fifteen minutes and was shocked when I arrived at the nursery. The patient was a six-pound newborn girl who had a quite pronounced omphalocele, accompanied by labored breathing. The nursery nurses had oxygen on her; she was not cyanotic (dusky, bluish skin color) but obviously wouldn't be able to sustain herself for long, struggling to breathe like that.

They had also covered her omphalocele with a wet, normal saline-soaked sponge. Fortunately, I had brought a complete set of state-of-the-art newborn endotracheal tubes and laryngoscope blades with me from Minneapolis and the nurses got them ready to go. As I prepared to intubate the baby, I told the nurses to call Minneapolis for their air ambulance to come get our little girl ASAP and also to coordinate with the University of Minnesota to have a neonatologist come with them. Intubating her was no problem, and after securing the endotracheal tube well and listening to her chest to make sure both lungs were being adequately ventilated, I proceeded to ventilate her with a baby AMBU bag.

Now we had another situation. We didn't have a ventilator in the hospital, let alone one suitable for pediatric use. That meant I would have to hand-ventilate her for as long as it took for the emergency crew to arrive from Minneapolis—and the average respiratory rate for a newborn is around forty-five breaths per minute. The air ambulance had estimated they could be there in about five hours.

I sat on a comfortable chair, rested my arms on a pad on the side of the bassinet, and started ventilating her. I could only keep up the pace for about fifteen minutes per hand. After an hour of that, I showed one of the nursery nurses how to do it so she could relieve me for a while. The baby's color was nice and pink, and her heart rate remained stable. We were confident we were doing a good job and that she'd be fine. It was exhausting work. Both of us had aching arms and hands by the end of our turn.

As luck would have it, the air ambulance arrived in almost five hours to the minute and brought a very nice young lady, a senior neonatology resident, with them. She took one look at the situation and marveled at our ingenuity. She was also very impressed when she saw the type of endotracheal tube that had been used. She told me that ordinarily, in cases like these, she would have to reintubate the infant because of the type of endotracheal tube in the baby, but due to the situation she just swapped out the one that she'd brought with her for the one I'd used.

There was a waiting ambulance outside the ER. After transferring our baby to a portable incubator, we brought our little girl's mom in to speak to the doctor and say her tearful goodbyes. They were gone in an hour, and my "nurse ventilating partner" and I were left exhausted. My arms felt like I'd been lifting weights all day. I went to the cafeteria for breakfast and then home to bed. Four hours later I got a call from the nursery to tell me that the neonatologist had been in contact with them, reporting that all was well and that the baby was in their neonatal ICU on the ventilator. Discussions about surgery for her were already underway.

What a comforting feeling.

I entertained the thought of how to approach our hospital administrator about purchasing two ventilators, one for newborns and one for adults. It would be two more years before we added a respiratory therapist to the staff and that happened.

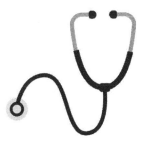

79. Too Fat

One morning my first patient for a colonoscopy was a sixty-seven-year-old woman who was only five feet tall and weighed four hundred pounds. She was diabetic and hypertensive, both under control with medication, and other than her morbid obesity she was relatively stable. Her diagnosis: history of chronic constipation.

Colonoscopies were done in the endoscopy department on a surgical stretcher with the patient lying in the lateral dorsal recumbent position. The usual anesthetic for colonoscopy is monitored anesthesia care (MAC), whereby the patient is sedated to effect for whatever maneuvers the gastroenterologist needs to accomplish. Depending on the patient's health status, body mass index and level of anxiety, several anesthetic agents may be used individually or in combination to achieve optimal sedation.

When I spoke to the lady in preop, she was very congenial and amenable to this type of anesthetic, since she'd had it before without any problems. I gave her a small IV dose of tranquilizer (Versed), and we brought her to the procedure room. I hooked up all the anesthesia monitors and had low-flow oxygen running to her via nasal cannula. She lay on her left side with her right arm bent at the elbow and her right hand—with the IV cannula in it—up by her chest for easy access. I sat on a stool about two feet in front of her face, so I could keep a close watch on her respirations and administer incremental doses of anesthetic agents to her through the IV. The gastroenterologist and his assistant were on the other side of the patient standing opposite me. I started injecting Propofol into her IV and, when she drifted off to sleep, I gave the team an okay to start.

The doctor and I were friends and the procedure was going smoothly, so we passed the time with some light conversation. At one point, during the procedure, I mentioned to him, "Do you ever tell these patients that one of the reasons they have problems like this is because they're so damn fat?"

With that the lady's eyes snapped wide open. Looking directly at me, she said in a slurred voice, "Was that comment directed at me?"

That shocked me. She was tolerating the procedure so well that I thought she was well anesthetized. Our conversations ended abruptly, and I hurriedly gave her a little more Propofol and added another dose of Versed. I hoped that would give her amnesia so she'd wake up with no recollection of my callous remark.

The rest of the case went smoothly and silently—except for conversation directly related to the procedure—and at the end of it our patient woke up nicely. I told the recovery room nurses what had happened and asked them to call me immediately if the lady said anything about it. Thankfully, she made no mention of anything related to my remarks, and they never called.

The incident prompted gales of laughter in the staff room for a long time afterward.

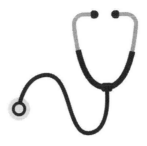

80. Skin Wheal

As I've mentioned, regional (either spinal or epidural) is the anesthetic of choice for elective cesarean section. That way, the unborn baby doesn't get any of the depressant effects of general anesthetic drugs in the mother's bloodstream.

One morning in the early 1990s, my assignment was to cover OB. The one lady in labor then wasn't progressing, so her doctor decided to do a cesarean section. The patient was a tall, thin, young gal and this was her first baby. She also was a single mother and didn't have anyone with her. She had been laboring for quite a while, so her doctor didn't want to wait for an epidural and opted for a spinal anesthetic, which works much faster. The lady was fine with that choice.

To administer a spinal anesthetic, I usually had my patient sitting up on the edge of the OR table facing away from me with the circulating nurse holding her in position. After prepping the back and locating my landmarks, I would make a 1 cc skin wheal of 0.5 percent xylocaine from a tuberculin syringe with a 27-gauge needle, at the appropriate level, effectively numbing the skin before I inserted the larger spinal needle. After that, depending on the patient's size, I'd insert the spinal needle approximately three centimeters through the numb area to reach the spinal canal and deposit the anesthetic mixture.

My patient was sitting comfortably on the edge of the OR table, resting her head on the shoulder of the circulating nurse, who was standing in front of her holding her steady. Her obstetrician was in the hallway at the scrub sink getting ready. We were all having a nice chat, and when I finished washing her back with prep solution, I told her that she'd feel a little needle stick as I numbed a spot on her back. I inserted just the tip of my 27-gauge needle just under her skin and injected the 0.5 percent xylocaine local anesthetic. No sooner had I finished than she let out a loud gasp and yelled, "*Oh, Oh. Oh, Heavens. I'm going to faint!*"

I instantly pulled the needle out of her back, grabbed her, and told the circulator to help me get her lying flat. Once we got her down, she felt much better. Her blood pressure had dropped a bit, but the rest of her vital signs were stable. Next, she told me that her legs and lower abdomen were getting numb. I tested those areas. Sure enough, she was profoundly numb, as though I'd actually injected into her spinal canal. I yelled to her obstetrician, "Get the hell in here, quickly. I think I just accidentally gave your patient a spinal doing the skin wheal. And I was only using a little bit of .5 percent xylocaine, so you don't have much time, because this stuff doesn't last long."

The doctor rushed into the room, and we had the patient prepped and draped in a flash. She tested the patient's skin and proceeded with the incision. The doctor had a healthy baby boy out and in the nursery bassinet in less than five minutes. Closing up the lady's belly took another fifteen minutes and by the time the dressings were on, my patient was starting to be able to wiggle her toes and get sensation in them. When we got her back to her room she had recovered completely, with minimal discomfort. I repeated to her some words I'd heard once from a famous surgeon after a carotid case: "All's well that ends well."

I discussed this case later with my colleagues. None of them had ever heard of the membrane covering the spinal canal being that close to the skin's surface. It was obviously a rare anomaly that I probably should have written up and submitted to an anesthesia journal.

I had a long talk with the patient about it for possible future surgeries and cesarean sections, and I recommended that she get a neurological consult and medical alert bracelet. I also had a meeting with the OB department staff to have them reinforce my suggestions to her.

I hope she took my advice.

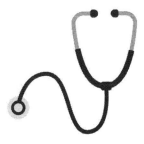

81. The Observer

On a beautiful northern-country Saturday afternoon in 1980, my wife and I were downtown shopping. I was on call that day and heard my beeper go off. We were close to the hospital so we both went there to see what was happening. There was an elderly, frail little lady who had just come into the ER with a broken hip that needed to be fixed. These cases should be done as soon as possible, since allowing a patient like her to lay inactive in a hospital bed for very long leaves her at risk for a potentially fatal case of pneumonia.

The type of hip fracture she had was one that, in those days, was fixed by replacing the ball portion of the thigh bone that fits into the hip socket of the pelvis. This operation didn't take very long and my wife decided to wait for me. I thought it might be fun for her to come into the OR and watch the case, since she'd never seen surgery firsthand before. She thought so too, so I asked the surgeon for approval and he was okay with it.

In those days most hip fracture cases on the elderly were done under spinal anesthesia. Fortunately, this lady was relatively healthy for her age so, after looking over her chart, I expected her to tolerate the anesthetic and procedure well.

We brought our lady to the OR and while I hooked up the monitors and got her spinal anesthesia in place, so she'd be numb from her lower chest on down, the circulating nurse got my wife outfitted in a scrub suit, mask, and hairnet. After our patient was prepped and draped, the nurse brought my wife into the OR to stand on a stool next to me so she could see over the drapes and watch everything. Because of our patient's advanced age, I hadn't sedated her

211

much and she was comfortable lying on her side lightly dozing as the operation progressed.

At one point during the procedure, to my wife's surprise, she opened her eyes, looked up and said, "Is that me they're pounding on?" A little while later, when the surgeon popped the new titanium ball into her hip socket, blood droplets splattered out of the incision and all over the surgeon and his assistant's face (they didn't wear face shields in those days). My wife looked horrified! As the case was winding down and the surgical team started to close the incision, the little lady began to wretch so I grabbed a catheter and suctioned about 25 ccs of light-green bile out of her mouth and into the clear plastic canister by the anesthesia machine. My wife took one look at that and the color drained from her face and I thought she might faint. I called the circulator to quickly grab her, take her to the lounge and have her sit down with her feet up. After she left, the surgeon chuckled and said, "I'm surprised anything bothers her after living with you."

When the case ended, and after I took our lady to the recovery room, I found my wife sitting in the lounge in her street clothes sipping orange juice. The only comment she made was, "I don't know how anybody could do that kind of work. The green stuff in the suction bottle looked like pus to me."

She never wanted to watch another surgery again.

We still laugh about it to this day.

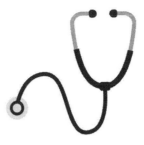

82. The Rebreathing Bag

In late 1969 I was a SRNA (student registered nurse anesthetist) with only a few months experience and in my first rotation at a large trauma and teaching center in downtown Minneapolis. Their daily surgery schedule varied from small, short cases all the way to kidney transplants and brain surgery, and there were students from every area of medicine and level of experience working together regularly. As a student, I always had a staff CRNA directing me although many times they'd remain just for the start of the case and then be available only if you called them after that. There was always an anesthesiologist somewhere in the department, but they were usually teaching their own residents, so we didn't work with them much.

One morning, the first case in my room was a ventriculoperitoneal shunt on an eighteen-month-old otherwise healthy baby. This procedure is done for hydrocephalus to relieve the intra-cerebral pressure caused by excess fluid accumulation in the brain's ventricles. To accomplish this, a narrow piece of tubing is inserted into a cerebrospinal fluid-filled ventricle in the brain. The tubing is then passed under the skin and down into the abdomen where the fluid drains and is absorbed. These operations typically took about three hours and were usually performed by the chief resident with a few of his juniors helping him. An attending neurosurgeon was nearby but hardly ever present.

I was really nervous about doing the case. Although I'd read everything I needed to know about it, the thought of "inexperienced me" in charge of a baby's anesthetic for brain surgery made me almost want to quit the program.

I brought the little twenty-three-pound crying girl to the surgery suite in my arms. She was a real cutie pie with blonde hair and blue eyes and her mom and dad were crying when I took her from them. We used a different breathing circuit on the anesthesia machine for pediatric anesthesia and the breathing hoses, face mask, and rebreathing bag were much smaller than the adult ones and I had everything changed out and was ready to go. When I put her on the OR table on a warming blanket, my supervising CRNA quickly put a pediatric blood pressure cuff on her arm and taped my precordial stethoscope to her chest. Meanwhile, I placed a mask lightly on her face and had her breathe a mixture of halothane vapor and 100 percent oxygen.

Because of her crying, she went to sleep quickly. Once she was asleep, I intubated her and secured the endotracheal tube in place, while the CRNA started her IV and inserted a rectal temperature probe. Then the circulating nurse put a catheter in her bladder. Now we were all set to go. The OR table was turned ninety degrees, so the surgeon would have unobstructed access to her head, and she was prepped and draped. The thinking those days was to keep brain surgery patients—especially pediatric ones—breathing spontaneously and assist their respirations with your hand on the rebreathing bag, occasionally squeezing in rhythm with their respiratory rate. It was another measure of anesthesia depth and possible brain impairment.

Once the case was underway it went smoothly. The baby's heart rate and respirations were regular, and her IV was running well. Through my earpiece, attached to the precordial stethoscope on her chest, I noted that her breath sounds were clear. It was a best-case scenario. I monitored her IV fluid intake closely and had a mini-drip attached to a burette in line from the IV fluid bag. I would only let 10 ccs drip in at a time, and when the burette was almost empty, I'd refill it with another 10 ccs. I had calculated that her fluid needs would be 30-40 ccs/hour.

After about an hour into the case I stood up to let another 10 ccs into the burette but, as I reached back for the rebreathing bag, I realized it was gone! Immediately I had an awful, fear-filled, adrenaline-rush feeling. To make matters worse, I didn't even have an adult bag in the room because the CRNA had taken all that stuff out when we changed the machine over for pediatric use. I frantically looked all around; it was nowhere to be seen.

I had the circulator get on the overhead page system and call anesthesia STAT to my room. As my CRNA came running in, I yelled to him that I'd lost the rebreathing bag and needed another one immediately. He glanced over at a far corner of the OR, behind the head of the table and discovered it lying there against the wall. The bag was not a new one and not disposable and had probably been used many times, which had evidently stretched out the bushing in the narrow top end neck of the bag where it fit onto the yoke of the anesthesia machine and made the connection quite loose. It had coincidently fallen off when I stood up, while at the same time the circulating nurse had walked behind me to get something. In the hustle and bustle of the case, she'd kicked it into the corner without realizing it.

My CRNA snatched it up, wiped it off, and had it back in place immediately. Disaster averted! Strangely enough, nobody from the surgical team even seemed to notice my dilemma which was fine with me. Fortunately, the baby was breathing spontaneously so she was never without oxygen. With the rebreathing bag gone, however, there was a massive leak in the circuit which diluted the anesthetic gasses and if left unchecked for very long it would cause her to wake up in the middle of the case. That never happened.

I was relieved, but my nerves were jangled, and I asked the CRNA to give me a break so I could go collect myself. After a half hour, two glazed donuts, a cup of black coffee, and a potty stop I settled down and was ready to go back. I brought another pediatric rebreathing bag with me just to be safe.

The rest of the case went well and uneventfully. At the end of it, the cute little girl woke up fine but wasn't happy. She cried loudly until we brought her mother into the recovery room. As a famous surgeon told me recently, "All's well that ends well."

I can still see everything about that situation in my mind to this day.

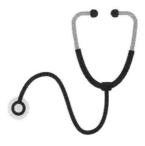

83. Lawsuit and Expert Witness

When I moved to Florida in 1987, I joined a mixed group of seven anesthesiologists and twelve CRNAs. We covered two hospitals with a total of eight operating rooms and one obstetrics department. The types of cases we did in the OR ranged from simple procedures to neurosurgical and thoracic surgeries and everything in between.

In early 1995, I received a certified letter from a firm of local attorneys informing me of their intent to file a lawsuit against me and my attending anesthesiologist over a case we had done a year before. The case alleged that our patient had suffered vocal cord damage from my intubation of her. I had no recollection of that case, but when I pulled her chart from the archives and looked at the anesthetic record and postop notes, I didn't see anything that indicated an airway problem before, during, or after the intubation or extubation.

Later that day, the firm of attorneys retained by our malpractice insurance carrier called me and explained that evidently my patient had developed a granuloma on one of her vocal cords a few months subsequent to the procedure. She had seen an ENT doctor who successively removed the granuloma and she was advised by him that it had been caused by her recent intubation—most likely, an inappropriately large-sized endotracheal had been used on her. That surprised me, because sizing the endotracheal tube to fit the patient was always one of my primary concerns in airway management. I always kept a selection of endotracheal tube sizes close at hand in the event that, upon direct laryngoscopy, the one I selected for the patient wasn't the right size. Our lawyer told me that the suit hadn't been filed yet and to just sit tight until it was.

A granuloma is a structure formed during an inflammation process and is found to be associated with many situations. It's a collection of immune cells (macrophages) that form when the immune system attempts to wall off substances it perceives as foreign but is unable to eliminate. On a vocal cord they may form as a response to irritation, such as from contact with an endotracheal tube. Anyone is at risk of getting a vocal cord granuloma and it is a known, remote possible side effect of short-term intubation.

My attending anesthesiologist and I scrutinized her chart looking for any indication of a postoperative airway issue, but we couldn't find a thing. However, one glaring omission stood out on the anesthetic record: Where the endotracheal tube size was supposed to be notated, there was no entry. I had forgotten to write it! I had no explanation for that glaring mistake and obviously that was the reason for this impending lawsuit. There was nothing to do now but wait.

Within a month, the suit was filed, asking for monetary compensation because of voice impairment due to the vocal cord granuloma suffered post-intubation from an allegedly inappropriately large-sized endotracheal tube. There was no denying the presence of the granuloma or the fact that the lady had been intubated or that she had suffered voice impairment. The issue all boiled down to what size the endotracheal tube was that she had been intubated with and if I had committed malpractice in using a larger size than was indicated for her. She was examined by an ENT doctor of our choosing, who pronounced her vocal cords normal now that the granuloma had been removed. However, the lady still claimed to have a hoarse voice and always wore a scarf around her neck, which our ENT specialist was convinced was a ruse to enhance the credibility of her lawsuit.

For the better part of 1995 the anesthesiologist and I gave depositions and had many conferences with our attorneys. At one point our insurance carrier offered her a cash settlement, which she promptly refused because she wanted a lot more money. Finally, with negotiations in a stalemate the case went to trial.

Six jurors, all handpicked by the attorneys, and a judge were assembled to hear our case. The plaintiff presented her case first and had as an expert witness the testimony of a retired anesthesiologist from Ohio. He was never present in the courtroom but claimed in a sworn deposition that the lady's vocal cord granuloma could only have occurred from being intubated by an inappropriately large-sized endotracheal tube.

After a couple days of the plaintiff's presentation our defense team was ready to go. My attending anesthesiologist testified first and was questioned about his role in supervising me, what procedures and guidelines were in place for oral intubation, and if he had been present during the induction and intubation phase of the case. After a day of that, it was my turn on the witness stand. The plaintiff's lawyer went first, and after the preliminaries regarding my credentials and experience (I had been practicing anesthesia for twenty-six years at the time), he started trying to portray me as callous and cavalier in my approach to his client's anesthetic.

He asked me things like, "How many endotracheal tubes do you have in your department?" and, "How many different sizes do you have immediately available on your anesthesia table in the OR?" "Where are they kept, and how far away from your OR were they at the time my client was on the surgery table?" "What criteria do you use in selecting the size of an endotracheal tube prior to intubating a patient?" "What kind of laryngoscope blade did you use to intubate my client with, and was it with your right or left hand?" "Here's a laryngoscope. Please demonstrate to the jury and explain just how you would normally use it in the course of intubating a patient."

At one point during my descriptive demonstration, the plaintiff's lawyer smugly attempted to interrupt me in an obvious attempt to distract my train of thought. I cut him off in the middle of his remarks by saying, "If you could possibly be courteous enough to let me finish, all your questions might be answered." He looked toward the bench, but the judge just told me to proceed with the testimony. Next, he asked me why I hadn't written the size of the endotracheal tube I had used to intubate his client in the correct place for it on the chart, suggesting that I had neglected to do so on purpose because I knew it was too large. I explained it was nothing more than oversight since I would never purposely do something like that. He turned, smiling to the jury, and said, "No further questions."

Next, our attorney took the line of questioning all through my training, career and expertise, dwelling on the fact that I had practiced anesthesia in a small rural hospital in northern Minnesota for sixteen years with only one other CRNA in the department to cover all the scheduled and emergency surgery cases. He also emphasized the point that "Mr. Whitchurch, after all his experience as an independent practitioner, would never put a wrong-sized endotracheal tube into a patient's airway." I hoped that resonated with the jury.

After all the direct and cross-examination was finished, it was time for the attorneys' closing remarks. The plaintiff's closing remarks were basically just a summation of the testimony and an attempt to impress the jurors with my negligence. When our attorney rose to speak, however, he was eloquent. He characterized us as excellent professional practitioners with sterling characters that would never, under any circumstance, employ a technique injurious to a patient. He had a small stack of anesthesia textbooks on the table in front of him and in closing he picked them up chest-high, saying, "If developing a granuloma on your vocal cord is not a known uncommon side effect of intubation and is instead malpractice, then why isn't it listed as such in any one of these textbooks?" On the word "textbooks" he slammed them all down on the table with a resounding bang like a rifle shot. The courtroom was silent for a moment before the judge instructed the jury, and they retired to deliberate.

Inasmuch as this was a civil trial and not a criminal one my attending anesthesiologist and I left the courtroom to go home. The attorneys stayed and it wasn't much more than an hour before the jury returned, exonerating us of malpractice. And the wonderful part of it was that the plaintiff gave up her right to appeal the verdict in exchange for us not bringing suit against her for the enormous cost of a year of litigation. What a huge relief!

Epilogue:

After that yearlong and nerve-wracking litigation experience, I decided to help other CRNAs who might find themselves in a similar situation. I told my attorney to call me if he ever needed an expert witness for the defense of another nurse anesthetist involved in a lawsuit.

One month later I received a call from his office asking me to review a case involving an arm board that fell off the OR table with an anesthetized patient's arm strapped to it. The type of arm board in question is one commonly used and is usually attached to the table after the patient is on it by a lip that fits over the top of the table's side rail and a hook that grabs the railing from underneath, making it secure. They are slightly cumbersome, weigh approximately five pounds, are well-padded and are easy to put on and take off the table. But if, for some reason, the lip and hook are not seated properly the arm board might look like it's attached properly but can actually be in such a precarious position that it could fall off at the slightest touch. That's why it's extremely important to test the integrity of that connection before strapping a patient's arm to it.

Responsibility for the placement of arm boards is shared between OR and anesthesia personnel. However, if the arm board is supporting the arm that has the anesthesia IV in it 90 percent of the responsibility to see that it's properly attached to the table falls upon the anesthesia provider. Such was the essence of this case. An arm board with an anesthetized patient's IV arm strapped to it was not securely attached to the OR table, and while the case was in progress, evidently someone bumped it causing it to fall off the table. That pulled the patient's arm severely backward, dislocating her shoulder.

A lawsuit was brought against the CRNA, and I was called in as an expert witness for the defense. I went with the attorney to the hospital and examined the OR table and arm board in question. They were the standard, widely used type both in a good state of repair. I didn't have to even read the depositions to know that it was pure negligence for the CRNA involved to not have made absolute sure that the arm board, with the arm and IV in it for administering all anesthetic drugs, was attached to the table properly and I told my attorney so as we left the building. His opinion was that it was not the CRNA's but the circulating nurse's responsibility to make sure the arm board was secure. That made me laugh. Then he suggested that I rethink my opinion, because he had a hospital manual from somewhere out of state that listed arm boards in the OR as the circulating nurse's responsibility. I told him that was a general rule and not specific to the circumstances of this case. He persisted with his nonsense, and when we reached his office I told him that no jury in the land would ever believe that and that he should call the insurance company today and tell them to pay the claim. My parting shot was: "If that happened to your wife or mother, you'd see this a whole lot differently."

I never heard any more about the case.

Another lawsuit in which I was called upon to defend a CRNA involved an epidural anesthesia catheter and the concomitant use of blood thinners.

Continuous epidural anesthesia is a type of regional anesthetic used for many lower extremity and abdominal procedures. It involves threading a small catheter through a special needle between the spinal vertebrae and into the epidural space—next to the spinal canal and separated by a membrane—through which local anesthetic is injected rendering the patient numb from their lower chest down to their feet. The epidural space is small and has many veins in it, so a catheter threaded into that area could traumatize the veins causing minor bleeding. This is usually self-limiting, causes no neurological symptoms, and resolves without medical intervention. However, if the use of an indwelling epidural catheter is associated with the administration of blood thinners, a complication called epidural hematoma may occur. This is serious because the effects of pressure from the hematoma can cause compression and ischemia of the spinal cord or nerve roots leading to neurologic sequelae, including paralysis. Such was the circumstance here.

An elderly lady received an epidural anesthetic during her surgical procedure to repair a hip fracture. Postoperatively, the epidural catheter was left in place for pain control, which is not uncommon, and attached to a pump metering in a continuous flow of low-dose local anesthetic. It's also a relatively common practice to put this type of patient on a blood thinner postoperatively so that a blood clot (deep vein thrombosis) doesn't develop possibly leading to blood clots in the lungs (pulmonary emboli) which is a critical condition.

Her surgery went well, and the lady was quite comfortable afterward with an epidural pump running. The orthopedic surgeon started her on blood thinners the second postop day but never communicated that information to the anesthesia provider and, evidently, the anesthesia provider never thought to ask about it. Over the course of the next few days, the lady's legs became progressively weaker to the point of paralysis and it was then that her epidural was discontinued. X-ray examination revealed the presence of a significant epidural hematoma and she was immediately taken to the OR to evacuate it. Her paralysis was permanent. A lawsuit followed, and I was contacted to be an expert witness for defense of the anesthesia provider.

There was no question about the cause of the paralysis. The issue centered on communication between the orthopedic surgeon and the anesthesia provider relative to the timing and use of a blood thinner postoperatively. The defense lawyer had done some research that made him think responsibility for instituting the anticoagulant in the presence of an epidural catheter was entirely the surgeon's. My considered opinion, after twenty-seven years as a CRNA at the time, was that it was incumbent upon the anesthesia provider to discuss the timing of postop anticoagulant therapy with the surgeon so as not to have this kind of terrible situation develop. The defense attorney disagreed.

Finally, after many months passed, I was called to give a deposition. After lots of questions by the plaintiff's attorney, he ended by saying to me, "Let me ask you something, Mr. Whitchurch. A lady comes into the hospital to have her broken hip fixed and afterward goes home paraplegic. Something was done that was wrong, wasn't there?" Defense expert witness or not, I answered, "Yes, there was." My attorney looked stunned! When we left the deposition, and before he could say a word to me, I told him that I was all through with this and added that he should never call me again.

I heard later that the case settled out of court. Thus ended my short career as an expert witness.

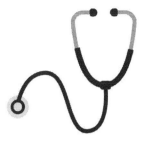

84. MH

Malignant hyperthermia is a disease condition defined as a severe systemic reaction triggered by certain drugs used in the administration of anesthesia. It is characterized by a fast rise in body temperature—up to 105 degrees or higher—severe muscle spasms, and a very rapid heart rate. Without prompt treatment the disease can be fatal. According to the National Institutes of Health, MH is inherited and only one parent has to carry the genetic predisposition for the disease for a child to inherit this condition.

Genetic testing and counseling is recommended for anyone with a family history of the disease. It occurs in one in fifty thousand to one in one hundred thousand individuals and may be more frequent than that because many people with an increased risk of this condition are never exposed to the drugs that trigger a reaction. The current treatment of choice for MH is administration of intravenous Dantrolene (first approved for MH use by the FDA in 1979) which is the only known antidote, along with immediate discontinuation of the triggering agents and supportive therapy directed at correcting hyperthermia, acidosis, and organ dysfunction. After the introduction of Dantrolene therapy the mortality rate of MH fell from 80 percent in the 1960s to less than 5 percent currently. Dantrolene still remains the only known drug to be effective in the treatment of MH.

In 1972, in our little hospital, one of the morning's first surgery cases was a seven-year-old girl named Alice for a scar revision on her neck. The scar was from an old tracheotomy she'd had at the University of Minnesota at age four because of a severe case of croup. She was a resident of the Red Lake Indian

Reservation and had been sent to the university by the public health hospital there for treatment.

The case was in my partner's room. After he'd made his preop assessment, he adjudged her to be very healthy and cooperative. Because it would be a relatively short case, he opted to do a halothane/oxygen inhalation induction of anesthesia and start her IV after she was asleep. That was a common technique for children and avoided the "dreaded needle stick." I was in another OR doing a short case and just as I finished it, I heard a lot of commotion in my partner's room. People were running in and out and yelling commands to each other.

As I passed by on the way to the recovery room with my patient, I asked what was going on. The circulator said that the little girl had a high fever and racing heart and that it was probably a malignant hyperthermia episode. As quickly as I could, I dropped off my patient and ran back to help. They had a rectal temperature probe in the little girl—which was showing 104.9—plastic bags of ice on her torso and legs, and were just hooking up some refrigerated saline to her IV. My partner said that right after the induction she started sweating profusely and her face was "on fire." He had quickly intubated her and was giving her 100 percent oxygen.

I ran to get what I needed to change out the granules in his carbon dioxide absorber canister, which were already turning blue, indicating that she was exhaling a lot of CO_2 and was probably quite acidotic. The granules also contained trace elements of the halothane my partner had been using which is a known triggering agent. The circulator got the iced saline running in her IV and another nurse put a urinary catheter in her. My partner and I alternated hyperventilating her in an attempt to get rid of the carbon dioxide building up from her acidosis. I changed the CO_2 granules one more time, and after forty-five minutes of this therapy, her temperature was down to 102.8, and she was making urine. It took another forty-five minutes to finally get her temperature down to 99.5. At that point, she started breathing on her own and waking up so we took the ice bags off her and changed out the IV fluid to room temperature.

Finally, cute little Alice woke up crying and we were so happy that everyone in the room cheered. My partner took her to the recovery room and we decided that she needed to stay the night in ICU. He also went out to discuss what had just happened with her parents and when he returned, he said that they were anxious, happy, and relieved. They also said that after the surgery she'd had at the university, they were told that she was a little slow to wake up. That definitely sounded to both of us like she may have had an episode of MH there, and either it wasn't explained well to the parents or they didn't understand. In either case, they had not followed up. He also told them that now she needed to wear a medical alert bracelet and that all the family members needed to be tested to see if they had the genetics for malignant hyperthermia.

Alice did well in ICU and was discharged home the next day after more instructions regarding MH.

She never got her scar revised.

Epilogue:

We had a meeting with the OR staff and director of nurses about MH a week afterward. It's a terrible complication of anesthesia and, although rare, there are case reports of patients dying from it. This was, however, the first one that our hospital and my partner or I had ever seen. He and I came up with a protocol for treatment should our hospital ever encounter such a case again.

Alice's case was a topic of discussion around our OR for a long time. Periodically, we'd receive notices of anesthesia seminars on MH and about a year after our incident, my partner decided to go to a weekend one at the University of Minnesota. When he came back from the seminar he laid a bombshell on all of us. After many lectures presenting didactic information the first day, the second day was all about case reports. He said that the very first case report was by an anesthesiology resident from the University of Minnesota, presenting a case from 1969 of a four-year-old girl from northern Minnesota with a severe case of croup sent to them for treatment by the public health hospital on the Red Lake Indian Reservation. He described how her respiratory distress became worse after she arrived, to the point of needing a tracheotomy. She was taken to the operating room, anesthetized, and the tracheotomy performed. Toward the end of the procedure she became quite diaphoretic and febrile. They quickly ended the procedure, applied ice to her trunk and legs, and administered chilled IV fluids. After an "extended" period of time her temperature normalized and all was well.

They characterized the incident as a relatively mild case of malignant hyperthermia. My partner was stunned to say the least. It was quite obvious that the case was our little Alice, who had the full-blown MH episode in our OR a year before. After the presentations were over, there was an informal gathering with all the lecturers and my partner was able to find the resident who presented Alice's case to let him know what had happened to her in Bemidji. He told me that he had tried not to be too confrontational with the fellow because it hadn't been his case, but it was hard to contain himself after the stress he'd suffered trying to save Alice's life, only to find out that it all could've been avoided had he known about her prior episode.

The resident had no explanation for how that could've happened. He told my partner that he would certainly check into it though. The worst of it was the fact that when Alice presented to us from the public health hospital for her scar revision, the chart that came with her made no mention of that incident at the university. My partner told me that just discussing the subject with a member of the anesthesia department there made his anger boil over to the extent that his last comment to the resident was that they were "Grossly negligent and it almost cost a little girl her life by not informing everybody, including her parents, about the incident. It should have been in big red letters on all her health records and this resident needed to tell his department head about it."

We never heard any more from the university. And I never had to deal with another case of malignant hyperthermia in my career.

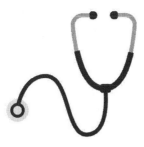

85. Mildred

"Mildred, I have something for you." These were the words a husband said to his wife before he pumped a slug point-blank into her liver on a Sunday evening in the late '80s.

I was at home and fortunately received a call from the hospital before she arrived, since the police had already notified them she was coming in and what the circumstances were, and I got to the emergency room about the time the ambulance arrived. The patient was a middle-aged woman, gasping, covered with blood and miraculously barely alive. We quickly got two large bore IVs into her arms and sent blood for lab work and a type and crossmatch, and I ran to the OR to get ready.

Our surgeon was a very talented young fellow who'd had plenty of trauma experience so when we got the lady on the OR table, I anesthetized her quickly and he didn't waste any time getting her belly open. Her abdomen was full of blood, which was running out of her and onto the floor. Meanwhile, because her blood pressure was extremely low from the blood loss, I had to give her universal donor type O negative blood until the type and crossmatches were finished. Our new anesthesia machine, which had a ventilator on it, freed up my hands to pump blood into her through both IVs.

I didn't have much time to do anything else except that, so I told a circulator to call the operator and have her get one of my partners in to help me out (at that time, we had three full-time CRNAs and one part-timer). My partner, a smart young gal with plenty of experience, came right in and for the next four hours all the two of us did was pump blood and push drugs. The lab called in all the donors they had with our lady's blood type, and the lobby was full of folks waiting to donate. Lab personnel also came in to help so they could keep up with everything. As soon as any blood was ready they sent it over—and it would still be warm from the donor.

Our surgeon and his assistant were working fast, trying to find all the bleeding points. The slug had ripped up a lot of tissue and it was coming from everywhere. He even had to resect part of her liver. That she was alive and tolerating all this was a testament to our surgeon's skill and the lady's resilience. Her blood pressure remained very low throughout surgery and, because of the massive blood loss, our circulators were changing out suction canisters frequently. Even with two of us pumping blood into each arm, we were barely able to keep up with it. As we'd finish one unit, we'd throw the empty bag into a box and quickly hang another one.

Finally, the case ended. The surgeon had stopped all her bleeding, resected her liver, and taken out her spleen and part of her bowel. Her vital signs were stable enough, although her blood pressure remained low, and we took her to ICU and put her on the ventilator. My partner and I were exhausted and I thanked her profusely for coming in because without her help the lady wouldn't have survived. We cleaned up our equipment, restocked our drawers, and got everything ready for another emergency case. A full box of empty blood bags remained unaddressed, but I was too tired to go through and chart them—all that could wait until morning. I went to ICU and checked on her once more before I left and she was still hanging in there.

The next morning, I went to see her right away. As I suspected might happen, Mildred died during the night. When I went back to the OR to chart the blood we'd given her, I counted forty empty blood bags. The average blood volume of a normal adult female is approximately four and one half liters, or nine units. That meant we had transfused her total blood volume over four times! Thank Heaven there were enough people in town with her blood type. At that time handling empty blood bags barehanded wasn't considered a bad idea, and when I was all done counting them my hands were bloody and sticky—something abhorrent by today's standards.

That was the last big case I ever did in Minnesota.

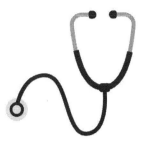

86. Nursery

One morning in 1991 I was assigned to work in the obstetrics department. They hadn't called needing anything at that point, but I thought I'd better go there to see if anything was pending. I took the stairs down one flight, which opened up to the hallway that had a window into the newborn nursery. It was full of cute babies and nurses bustling about tending to them. As I stood there watching, a young lady wandered over next to me to look in the window too. I assumed she came from the postpartum section of the department, because she was dressed in a hospital gown and bathrobe, had come from that direction, and looked the part.

As we stood there for a few minutes looking at the babies together, I turned to her and smilingly asked, "Which one of these little cuties is yours?" She gave me a horrified look, burst into tears and ran off. I was surprised to say the least. When I told one of the OB nurses about it, she said, "Oh, my god! You didn't say it to that lady, did you? She just had a stillborn baby yesterday." I really felt bad hearing that, but it had been an honest mistake on my part. Those patients are always transferred out of the OB department to the regular hospital ward to avoid being traumatized by the happiness of all the mothers and their newborns. She had wandered over to the nursery from there.

Obstetrics is an emotionally charged department. Better to keep your mouth shut there, which wasn't my strong suit.

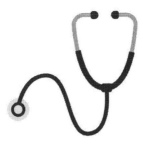

87. Multiple Personalities

One morning one of my patients was a lady in for a minor surgical procedure. She had another lady with her in the preop cubicle who was sitting on the chair next to her OR stretcher. After I introduced myself as the CRNA who would administer the anesthetic for her surgery, her friend spoke up first—and with a bit of an attitude.

"I'm her therapist, and I've been working with her for a long time and I just want you to know that she has multiple personalities, three of them! And I need to know which one you're going to put to sleep."

That put me off a bit, but after some quick thinking, I said to her, "Well, let's think about this for a minute. All of those personalities come from her brain, don't they?" She hesitated, glaring at me and trying to figure out where I was going with that remark. Finally, she agreed that they did, so I added, "I'm going to put her brain completely to sleep, so don't you think all the personalities will go to sleep too?"

She reluctantly had to agree, but vehemently added, "I insist on being in the recovery room when she wakes up, because they're all completely different people. I don't know which one will wake up and I'm the only one that knows who they all are."

I assured her that I'd make arrangements for that and asked her which personality I was talking to now? She said it was the one listed on her chart. For the rest of the interview, I spoke to the patient who was a very pleasant middle-aged lady. After I left, I alerted the head nurse in the recovery room to the situation, which gave her a good chuckle.

The case went well and when we got to the recovery room, there was her therapist dressed in a scrub suit waiting for her. I lingered a bit, hoping that a raunchy biker chick or a queen of Egypt would wake up, but it was the same lady I'd put to sleep.

What a disappointment.

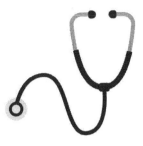

88. Faux Pas

Unlike these days, back in the '90s all surgical and obstetric patients were seen and interviewed privately by our anesthesia staff in the anesthesia office prior to their surgery or labor epidurals. That was usually an all-day assignment for a CRNA because of how busy those two departments were.

Late one morning, I had been interviewing mostly labor epidural patients and they usually had their significant other with them and it was always a happy time and cheerful interview. Most of them had been to prenatal classes, so our discussions centered on the mechanics of a labor epidural.

After seeing a string of pregnant ladies, a woman came into the office who appeared to be in the late stages of hers. She was familiar to me because she was an ICU nurse whom I knew casually from taking postop patients there. I greeted her at the office door with a big smile and said, "Good morning. Are you here to talk about your labor epidural?" There was a long pause and she replied with a scowl, "I'm not pregnant. I'm just fat!"

To say I was shocked would be an understatement and immediately anxiety welled up inside me. I hadn't looked at her paperwork before I said that to her, I had just made an assumption. I managed to stammer out a barely adequate apology that, of course, fell on deaf ears. When I finally did look at her preop papers I saw that she was there for back surgery. We sat across the desk from each other, her glaring at me, and me trying to regain composure and act pleasant. I was pretty sure my faux pas would get back to the chief of anesthesia, so I bore down on what few professional skills as an interviewer I could still muster.

Because she was a registered nurse from ICU and had seen many surgical patients, we didn't have to dwell much on the mechanics of her anesthesia. Mostly, we focused on what drugs she'd receive and how long the surgery would take, etc. I did most of the talking and she made a few curt replies. Thankfully, the interview didn't take long and she thanked me as she left by giving the office door a slam that sounded like a rifle shot.

I hurried to tell my chief what had just happened before he heard it through the grapevine. He said that was one of the best laughs he'd had in a long time.

I never worked with her in ICU again.

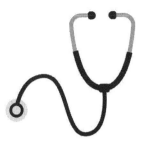

89. Speech Impediment

When I was young I learned how to whistle an "S" note through my front teeth, making it sound like I had a dental problem or a lisp and I'd do it really loud around family and friends as an attention-getting device and to get a few laughs. If I did it around a stranger, it was even funnier because they'd give me a strange look and try to ignore it probably thinking, "Oh, that poor man."

The mix of CRNAs and anesthesiologists I worked with in Florida was a pretty jovial group and one of the anesthesiologists, Jan Duvoisin, and I had the same offbeat sense of humor and we'd whistle Ss around each other frequently for a chuckle or two. He picked up on it quickly and, with a little practice, could do it very well too. Sometimes we'd sit and chat in the break room, whistling out all our Ss as we spoke.

One morning, while doing preop interviews in the office, one of my patient interviewees happened to be a very friendly middle-aged lady. We exchanged pleasantries and before discussing her anesthesia issues we socialized a bit. She had a cute sense of humor and after a few laughs we got down to business. She'd had surgery and anesthesia before without any complications and was healthy. As I looked over her chart and discussed the information with her, ever so slightly I let my whistled Ss creep into our dialogue. As I continued the discussion, I could see a quizzical expression forming on her face. When I got to her lab work, which was all normal, I really turned up the intensity of the whistles. Now she looked perplexed.

I said, "Let me check on thiSSS lab work with one of my SSSuperviSS-SorSSS and SSSee what he thinkSSS. It'll juSSSt take a minute." Now she was truly befuddled. I opened the door from the anesthesia office to the OR and—what a stroke of luck—Jan Duvoisin was standing right there.

I said, "Doctor DuvoiSSSin, could you pleaSSSe have a look at thiSSS lady'SSS lab work and SSSee what you think?"

He took her chart and said, with loud whistles, "YeSSS, I SSSee what you mean."

I turned to the lady and said, "We go to the SSSame dentiSSSt."

For a second she just looked shocked, then she burst into a huge laugh and so did Duvoisin and I. I told her that we'd been waiting for years for someone like her to come along so we could test our vaudeville routine. She said that it would be a huge success for sure.

That still ranks as one of the funniest highlights of my career. Jan Duvoisin and I still talk that way whenever we get together.

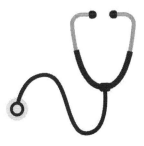

90. Graduate Student

My first case at one of the surgicenters that our anesthesia group covered was a knee arthroscopy on a pleasant middle-aged man. When I went to see him in preop, he was sitting up on the OR cart and had his pretty, young college-aged daughter next to him in a chair doing some work on a computer in her lap. After I finished explaining everything to the patient, I turned to his daughter and asked her if she was already doing schoolwork on her computer. She said, "Oh, yes, sir. I'm in graduate school at USF (University of South Florida), and we have a lot of work to do every day."

I commended her for her diligence and asked what she was studying. She replied, "I'm going to be a speech therapist, and we have to write a lot of papers." What an opportunity for me!

I replied, using my best lateral lisp, "ISSSh that SSSo? I have thiSSS friend who haSSS a bad liSSSp, and I wonder if that'SSS SSSomething you could fiXXX?"

She got a classic horror-film look on her face, and her dad laughed so hard he started coughing. Finally, she laughed too and so did all the nurses who heard me.

I'd been waiting for the opportunity to do that for a long time.

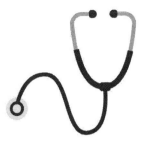

91. Rigid Bronchoscopy

Bronchoscopy is a procedure that allows a pulmonologist to have a direct look at the air passages inside your lung. During this procedure, a thin, flexible, fiber-optic tube is passed through your nose or mouth, then down through the throat and into your lungs. This procedure can be used to obtain samples of mucus or tissue, remove foreign bodies, or provide treatment for lung problems. Since the advent and perfection of fiber optics, most bronchoscopies are performed these days with heavy sedation type anesthesia and a topical anesthetic spray to the nose and throat, making it tolerable for the patient and the procedure to go smoothly.

Back in the late '60s, bronchoscopies weren't like that at all and were a real challenge for anesthetists. They were done under general anesthesia using a long, hollow, rigid, stainless steel tube with a light on one end and an eyepiece on the other, which was passed through the patient's mouth and down into their trachea and lungs. The bronchoscope had a side arm port on it to attach the connecter from our anesthesia machine hoses for delivering anesthetic gasses and oxygen to the patient. After the patient was asleep, a towel roll was placed under their shoulders, tilting their head backwards, and rubber guards were put over their teeth for protection. The rigid bronchoscope was then inserted through the mouth and down into their trachea.

To the casual onlooker, it was a brutal procedure and many a student nurse had to leave the room during it! The pulmonologist sat at the head of the table and had a large, round, plexiglass shield in front of his face fastened to a band around his head to protect him from any materials that might come spewing back up through the bronchoscope while he worked. An eyepiece was attached to the end of the scope, but when he needed to work through it, he'd take that off and pass long instruments down the scope to obtain specimens, to cauterize, and to suction bodily fluids.

It was difficult to ventilate the patient well under those circumstances because there wasn't a tight seal on the airway circuit, which always caused a substantial leak in it. Consequently, it was necessary to use high gas flows to keep the patient oxygenated and asleep. Also, even under general anesthesia airway reflexes are still relatively sensitive and occasionally the pulmonologist would elicit one causing the patient to have a somewhat diminished cough reflex. Also, the procedure was done in a darkened room so the surgeon could have better vision through the scope without ambient light interference. When everything was finished, the patients all had irritable throats and woke up with coughing fits that persisted well into their time in the recovery room. As you can imagine, none of the CRNAs liked doing these cases very much.

One morning as a three-month anesthesia student, the second case in my room at the hospital in Minneapolis was scheduled as a bronchoscopy with biopsies. I had done one before, which went well, but this one was on a very frail and sick elderly man with a big lung tumor. He had low hemoglobin, was short of breath, and looked cachectic. The doctor doing the case was a second-year thoracic surgery resident. I asked my supervising CRNA to give me a few pointers on how best to proceed with a patient this sick, and he said, "Just take it easy on him, and he'll do fine."

After our patient was asleep and positioned on the OR table, the lights went off and our thoracic resident began feeding the long, rigid bronchoscope into the old fellow's airway. I hooked my anesthesia hoses to the side arm so I could ventilate him and, in spite of all the leaks in the breathing circuit, the man's vital signs stayed stable.

Because the surgeon was a second-year resident, and this was a teaching case, he was taking his time examining structures and taking small bits of tissues as biopsies. Every so often he'd pull the scope out, clean the distal lens and reinsert it, making my attempts to keep the patient oxygenated a nightmare and also eliciting a significant cough reflex from the patient that was hard to control. I mentioned that to him once and only got a condescending glare with no response. I was anguishing and insecure over how long this case was taking and had a foreboding feeling that wouldn't go away. Also, it annoyed me that this resident was so seemingly overconfident and insensitive to my situation and to how delicately balanced and sick our patient was.

After an hour, the resident said, "I see where the tumor is and I want to get some pieces of it from all quadrants." That told me we were going to be there for quite a while longer. As he snipped out pieces of it, I squeezed the breathing bag vigorously and prayed he wouldn't take a bite out of any vital structure down there that might jeopardize and possibly kill this old man.

I didn't have to wait long because he got a hold of something down inside the patient's lung that made him struggle to snap the jaws of his long biopsy forceps shut and when they did, blood abruptly shot out of the end of the bronchoscope like a hose, hitting his face shield and splattering all over us. He pulled the forceps out, let out a loud gasp, and started shaking.

The circulating nurse yelled out, "Quick, pack the scope!"

I yelled out, "Call his attending!"

The surgeon put his finger over the end of the scope, wiped his face shield off, and started pushing rolled gauze sponges down the bronchoscope. That really didn't help. Blood was welling up around the scope from the trachea, filling the patient's mouth and spilling over onto the drapes, the floor, and me. It was impossible to ventilate him by squeezing the breathing bag because it would cause bubbles to come up through the blood, which would splatter it all over the place.

The patient's vital signs deteriorated rapidly. I could hear a very faint heartbeat, but his blood pressure was unobtainable. The attending thoracic surgeon arrived in about ten minutes, which seemed like an eternity and he didn't even ask what had happened; instead, he just looked at the scene and said, "I bet you got a piece of the pulmonary artery."

By then I couldn't hear a pulse, the patient's pupils were fixed and dilated and he was dead. The resident rolled his stool back with his head down, shaking it from side to side. His attending attempted to console him by saying, "This kind of thing happens occasionally." I had called my supervising CRNA to the room STAT and when he came in, he unleashed a string of epithets at how the room looked. When I told him what had happened, he stood there shocked said, "I always thought this guy was an overconfident resident."

There was blood running on the floor, splattered on all of us, on the overhead lights and even on the ceiling and I was fortunate not to have gotten any in my eyes because I wore glasses. The resident still sat on the stool with his head down as I took apart all my bloody anesthesia equipment. The room looked as though an axe murder had taken place.

A couple of orderlies took our patient to the morgue, one of the anesthesia aides came to help me clean up my equipment and a team of housekeepers cleaned the room. I went to the locker room and took a long, hot shower. There was even blood in my hair that had soaked through the surgery cap. I wished that my day had been finished after that disaster, but I had a bunch of smaller cases to do after that—and in the same room. Fortunately, they all went well but everywhere I looked, I thought I saw a drop of blood.

I had a long talk with the chief of anesthesia about that case, which he wanted me to write up to present at our monthly meeting. I did, but thankfully, I rotated to another hospital before I ever had to present it.

And I never worked with that resident again while I was there.

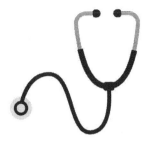

92. Ugly Doctor

Gastroenterologists do upper EGD (esophagogastroduodenoscopy) and lower (colonoscopy) endoscopic exams for many reasons. Some are routine, others are for ongoing pathological conditions and some are for critical/life-threatening issues. Almost all the routine and ongoing conditional exams are done in the GI (gastrointestinal) lab, with few exceptions. For ICU patients with critical health problems, most of which are GI bleeds, we have equipment on mobile carts so we can go to their room for the procedure.

One afternoon I was notified by the GI lab that they needed me to come to ICU for an EGD on an elderly man who was bleeding from his stomach because of the blood thinners he was receiving due to a recent MI (myocardial infarction—heart attack). When I arrived with my anesthesia cart, the GI lab crew was sitting around waiting for the doctor. Even though he had scheduled the case he had not seen the patient yet to introduce himself, discuss things, and get an informed consent signed for the procedure.

In a half hour, the GI doctor finally arrived with a thousand reasons why he was late. He was a good practitioner whom I'd worked with many times but had a quirky—and occasionally inappropriate—personality. I told him that he had to go see the patient and explain everything to him and his wife and get an informed consent from them because the ICU nurses told me the couple hadn't even been told that he would have the procedure. That shook the doctor up and he looked a little bewildered and stuttered out some lame excuse.

He and I went in to see the couple. The patient was a very frail old man who was hooked up to several IVs on pumps with two or three medications running in them. His wife was sitting in a chair next to him with a stern look on her face and she asked, "Who are you two and why are you here?"

The GI doctor, about as tactless as I've ever witnessed, introduced himself and said, "We're here to do a procedure and have a look in your husband's stomach with a scope to see if we can figure out why he's bleeding, and you'll have to leave the room for it."

The wife got a ferocious look on her face and said, "Over my dead body you will, and just who the hell do you think you are, anyway?"

That really left the doctor flustered and he started fidgeting trying to stammer out a reply. I had to suppress a chuckle and quickly left the room. After fifteen minutes, the doctor came out, obviously rattled, and announced that the wife had consented to let us do the procedure. I went in to talk to the couple about what kind of anesthesia I'd be using. They were very pleasant to me, though the lady couldn't help pointing out that our doctor was about as impertinent a fellow as she'd ever seen. I chuckled but didn't disagree with her.

The crew got set up, and the case was finally underway. The old man had two spots in his stomach that were oozing blood, so the doctor cauterized them through the endoscope, took some pictures, looked into the duodenum and in fifteen minutes we were done. He left the room to talk to the patient's wife while I woke the patient up and the GI lab folks cleaned their equipment. When I left the room I went to talk to the wife and, after I explained everything I had given him and how long it would be before he was fully awake, she said to me, "I have to tell you something. That doctor is about the ugliest man I've ever seen in my life! And I don't mean his personality, which is ugly too."

That made me laugh out loud, but I didn't say a word.

Our doctor needed a lot of work on his bedside manner.

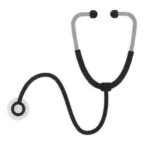

93. An Alcoholic's Cure

Esophageal varicies are abnormally enlarged veins in the esophagus. This condition occurs most often in people with serious liver diseases, such as scarring from cirrhosis—a relatively common occurrence in chronic alcoholism. The scarring cuts down on blood flowing through the liver; as a result more blood flows through veins of the esophagus. The extra blood flow causes these veins to balloon outward and can cause them to leak or possibly rupture, creating a life-threatening bleeding situation. Upon endoscopic exam, if any look to be at risk for rupturing, an elastic band is placed around them to cut off blood flow through the vein. The banded tissue quickly heals after several days and the procedure is safe, doing no damage to the esophageal wall.

I was working with my favorite gastrointestinal specialist one day in the GI lab, a very pleasant, intelligent and compassionate fellow who was quite adept at doing complicated procedures remotely through the endoscope. He also donated lots of his time to a free clinic in Florida to help the many poor and destitute souls there with their health problems.

After completing several cases on healthy people for routine follow-up procedures, he had a middle-aged lady patient with advanced alcoholic cirrhotic liver disease and esophageal varicies that needed to be examined with the endoscope to determine their fragility. My preop discussion with her was very pleasant and she was quite candid about her alcoholism, telling me all about the years of drinking and volume of her regular consumption. Amazingly though, she had stopped drinking and been sober for a year but, unfortunately, was suffering from the ravages of it now. She had been through many procedures like this and confessed that she had a great deal of remorse for how she'd ruined her health, shortened her lifespan and traumatized her family.

After taking her to the procedure room and anesthetizing her, the doctor slowly introduced an endoscope into her esophagus. He had scoped her six months before and banded some varicies, but from the looks of it many had reformed. As he was working, I mentioned our preop discussion to him and how amazed I was over the fact that considering how bad of an alcoholic as she had been, she could just all of a sudden stop drinking. I asked him if he knew what made her quit.

"I sure do," he replied. "She's been my patient for a long time and been drinking for years and getting progressively more cirrhotic every time I saw her. She would even come into my office drunk sometimes. Nothing I could do or say to her seemed to register enough to make her stop. The last straw was when she came to see me about a year ago and was really drunk. I was fed up with her by then, and I told her, 'Get out of my office! I never want to see you again! If you won't quit drinking, just go home and die! You're killing yourself, so get out of here and go do it!'"

Pretty strong words from the mild-mannered, compassionate guy I knew. I was amazed he had talked like that to a patient and told him so. I also told him that he might have the magic touch and should advertise a quick cure for alcoholism. He told me that she might have been the worst alcoholic he'd ever had as a patient.

He banded three or four of her esophageal varicies during the case and told me that because of her damaged liver, these would keep recurring and we'd have her back here frequently. She woke up fine and thanked us all profusely.

What a success story…all thanks to some harsh words.

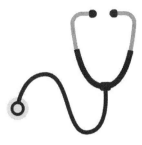

94. Donor

On a pleasant midsummer Thursday afternoon in the late '70s, the ER notified me that an ambulance was on the way with a girl who had sustained a possible head injury from a motorcycle accident. I had just finished the last case of the day in the OR, so I decided to go to the ER and see how she was. When they arrived, I noticed that the patient was a pretty, young college girl who was awake and alert, covered with bruises and scrapes and had a nasty bump on her head.

Evidently, she had been riding a little scooter without a helmet on the busy main street when a car pulled out in front of her. She ran into the side of it, flew over the hood, bumped her head when she landed and skidded about ten feet. That she was awake and alert was a good sign. Her pupils were equal and reactive, her vital signs normal, and all the rest of her neuro checks were fine. She wanted to go home, but the doctor and I were of the opinion that because of the big bump on her head, we needed to keep her for at least twenty-four hours for observation. She didn't like it but reluctantly agreed. The girl was admitted to a private room right next to the nurse's station adjacent to the OR so they could watch her.

The next morning, before the surgery schedule, I went to check on her. She wasn't awake yet but the nurse said she'd had a good night and hadn't complained about her frequent wake-ups for neuro checks. After my first case finished, I went to check on her again and found her sitting up, eating breakfast and in good spirits. She still had a bad headache and understood why she need-ed to be observed. When the doctor on duty came in, I asked him how long he planned to keep her. He said that all things being equal, and if she developed no bad symptoms from her head bump, probably until later that evening.

Periodically, between cases, I'd look in to check on her and she was always fine. When the surgery schedule was over, I checked on her one last time before I went home and the nurses told me that since nobody could stay with her where she lived, she had to wait until her parents arrived from Minneapolis before they would discharge her. They arrived in the late afternoon and were staying at a motel close to the hospital.

At five o'clock the next morning, I got a call from her doctor telling me that over the course of the evening she had become drowsy and that by midnight she was barely arousable. Now it was morning and she was unconscious, with labored breathing and one pupil fixed and dilated. He said that he had also called her parents and that I better come in to see if she needed to be intubated.

When I got there, both of her pupils were fixed and dilated, and her breathing was quite labored. The EEG (electroencephalogram) technician was on her way to do a "brainwave" test on her and the doctor had spoken to her parents about her condition. I got my equipment and quickly intubated her, which was easy because she had no airway reflexes. After that, her breathing improved, and I hooked up oxygen to her endotracheal tube. Her vital signs remained stable, although her pulse was very slow. The EEG technician arrived at 6:30 a.m. and quickly did an electroencephalogram on her. The results were not good. The doctor reluctantly pronounced her brain-dead.

That was a terrible blow to the girl's parents. At least when they arrived, she had been awake enough to know that they were there and have some meaningful conversation with them. Now, the doctor's discussion with her parents centered around their interest in donating her organs. After much soul-searching, they decided to go ahead with it.

At 7:30, the doctor called Minneapolis about the girl's situation and was told that they would send a team to us by noon to "harvest" her heart. I had never done a case like this before but the doctor said that they'd tell me everything I needed to know when they got there. I went to check on her once more before I got set up. Nothing had changed. Her vitals were stable and she was breathing on her own through the endotracheal tube. The supervisor called the OR crew in to get ready for our case, and after I got all set up, I went to the cafeteria for some breakfast and then to the staff lounge to wait.

A little after noon the team from Minneapolis arrived. They / plane and arrived at the hospital with their equipment in a van escorted , enforcement. The girl's doctor and I met them in the ER. They were a congenial group, comprised of a surgical team for the procedure and some social service staff to tend to legal issues and all the family's concerns. The thoracic surgeon and his assistant were very nice guys and when I told them that I had never done one of these before, they said that the main thing I needed to be concerned with was keeping the patient well-oxygenated and the blood pressure up by whatever means I had until they were ready to clamp the aorta and remove the heart. When they got to the OR, their nurses explained to our staff what was going to happen and the social services ladies went to talk to and be with the family. The doctors were impressed with our small surgery suite and told us that once they got started the whole procedure wouldn't take much more than an hour and a half.

The circulating nurse and I went to get our patient and after a tearful farewell from the family, which choked me up a bit, we brought her to surgery. By now her breathing was so shallow that I had to assist it with an AMBU bag. It was a very busy yet strangely subdued atmosphere in the OR and there was a lot of talking but no extraneous chatter, akin to a well-organized military operation. The team had their own scrub nurses and instruments, but one of our staff scrubbed in to help them. There were also two fellows to handle the harvested heart and two nurses to take care of the charting and paperwork. The social services ladies stayed with the family.

When we had her all prepped and draped, the doctors worked fast. Once the chest was open they did quite a bit of dissection to free up the heart from surrounding tissue. It was like a regular case to me at that point, but as they worked I had to use frequent doses of vasopressors (blood pressure medications) to keep her blood pressure up. Finally, the moment arrived to clamp the aorta and the surgeon alerted everybody, like a field commander. He clamped and cut the aorta, and his assistant lifted the heart out, quickly taking it to one of the waiting fellows who was gowned and gloved and had a sterile bag open to accept it. At that point my work was done. With mixed emotions I turned off the anesthetic gasses and watched them close the incision. When they were through, the team cleaned their instruments and left almost as quickly as they'd arrived, taking off to the airport in their waiting van where their plane was revved up and ready to go.

There was a lot of discussion among us while we were cleaning up. Everybody was glad to have had the experience, but the sad situation surrounding it was difficult for a few. A week later, the hospital nursing staff had a meeting about our case on the premise that it could happen again at any time and what everybody needed to know. The nurses that were there that day and I presented the case, with a lot of discussion afterward. Sentiments were all positive since a person with a sick heart was now going to get a new one and, thereby, a new life.

We never heard any details of who the recipient of the young woman's heart was.

Epilogue:

I have purposely omitted specifics relative to names, dates, organizations, and identifying location—except for our hospital, for obvious reasons. I also carefully avoided any details of the emotionally charged atmosphere and drama that existed for the same reasons.

Since I've been in Florida, I have been involved in a few more harvestings in which the team also took kidneys, liver, corneas, and long bones from the donor.

Nothing compares to the first time in that little hospital in northern Minnesota.

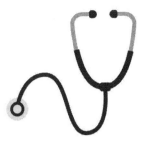

95. Three Veterinary Stories

I have a good veterinarian friend who lives in Bemidji. He had a very busy practice that he ran out of the lower level of his large house on Lake Bemidji. His surgery and office was state-of-the-veterinary-art and even had a small anesthesia machine with vaporizers and a ventilator on it, just like ours at the hospital. I used to go over to his place many days after my shift at the hospital was done to help him out and sometimes we'd even go on country calls together to take care of large animals, which was a lot of fun. His wife was his very savvy veterinary technician.

I really enjoyed the break from hospital routine. For almost every surgery he performed on small animals he would do an inhalation anesthetic induction. If it was a dog or cat, he'd fit a cone-shaped mask over their muzzle and then, if the surgery required it, intubate them after the induction.

One afternoon I planned to be his anesthetist during the spaying of a cat. I had watched him anesthetize small animals many times and was anxious to try it. He held the kitty while I blew anesthetic vapors mixed with oxygen across its face. When she was finally asleep enough to be intubated, he held her head for me so I could slip a little endotracheal tube into her trachea, and I got it on the first try. After that we positioned the kitty so he could do the spay and I monitored the character of her breathing and heart rate to gauge her depth of anesthesia.

The surgery went well and didn't take long, and soon it was time to wake the kitty up. Drawing on my experience from waking up humans, I turned the anesthetic vapors off and let her breathe straight oxygen for a while to get rid of them. When I saw her swallow a couple of times I decided she was awake enough to remove the endotracheal tube. I reached down to her mouth and grasped the endotracheal tube with my thumb and first finger, touching her nose in the process, which was evidently just enough stimulation to elicit a fierce bite reflex in her half-awake state. She clamped down on my thumb like a vise, hard enough for her fang to go right through my thumbnail.

Of course my first reflex was to jerk my hand up, and when I did it lifted her right off the table—while still attached to my hand. Not only that, it was also so excruciatingly painful that I let out a long string of profanities, evoking gales of laughter from my friend and his wife. He quickly came over and pried the kitty's mouth open so I could extricate my thumb, and then the kitty woke up. I soaked my thumb in some antiseptic solution and put ice on it and he gave me a few antibiotic pills to keep it from getting infected, with the admonition that after I took them I shouldn't be surprised if I develop a desire to use the sandbox instead of a toilet and that I might crave a steady diet of sardines for a while.

He also said, "Now, you're an official member of the Friends of Veterinarians Society for receiving your first certified animal bite in the line of a therapeutic endeavor."

On another occasion, I accompanied my friend on a country call to geld (castrate) a stallion that the farmer was having a hard time controlling. He told me having a veterinarian do it is the humane way to geld a horse; that way they get an anesthetic for the procedure. Unfortunately, some farmers used painful and inhumane ways to avoid a fee. I was to be the anesthetist and that way the hired man would hold the horse's bridle and the farmer could watch the surgery.

When we arrived, the farmer and hired man had the horse in a pasture next to the barn with his bridle tied to a lead rope attached to a steel post. He was a beautiful big chestnut stallion who stood sixteen hands tall with three white stockings and white blaze on his forehead. My friend had been to this place many times over the years and knew the farmer well and he introduced me as his anesthesia specialist who helped him occasionally. Next, he cautiously approached the stallion while holding out his hand for the horse to get his scent. My friend spoke in low, reassuring tones to the horse and was finally able to approach him and pet his forehead and nose.

The practice vehicle was near the pasture, so he and I went to get all the equipment and drugs we'd need. He explained that the hired man would hold the horse's bridle while he approached him from the front, eased around to the side, found the vein in his neck and then quickly injected it with Surital, a short-acting barbiturate. He would leave the needle in place and attach another syringe of Surital to it, which I would hold in case the horse needed more while he was working. Then he and the farmer would stand on either side of the stallion, and the hired man would hold his head to guide him to the ground and protect him from injury as he became unconscious. It sounded pretty simple.

We all got in position and my friend slowly approached the horse, holding his left hand out and speaking to him in low tones again. In his right hand, which he had concealed behind his back, he held a 50-cc syringe of Surital with a big needle on it. The horse sniffed his hand and let him rub his nose and head while my friend slowly moved to the side of the horse's neck. While petting him on the neck, my friend palpated it with his fingers at the same time and when he found the spot he was looking for, he gave the neck a light smack and then quickly inserted the needle there, injecting the whole syringe of Surital.

Almost immediately, the stallion's eyes shut, his head began to droop and his front legs started to buckle. As he was falling forward a bit, the hired man kept a firm grip on his head, and my friend gently pushed him toward the farmer so that he'd go down on his side. He went down gently on a soft, grassy spot. The hired man was still holding his head so he could breathe easily, and I had the syringe of Surital that was in his neck firmly in my hand. The veterinarian and farmer were at his hindquarters.

My friend worked quickly. He washed the stallion's scrotum with antiseptic solution, made an incision and clamped the spermatic cords. As he did this, the horse groaned and twitched a little. "Ron, give him half that Surital you have," he instructed me, then he cut the spermatic cords, took out the testicles and threw them over in the grass.

The farmer saw that, chuckled and said, "Doc, don't be so rough. Around here, them're quite a delicacy."

That made me laughed so hard, I almost pulled the syringe out of the now gelded animal's neck. When it was finished, I pulled the needle and syringe out of the horse's neck and held pressure on it for a few minutes. The whole operation took about fifteen minutes and we all waited around for another half hour to make sure our patient woke up safely. The horse opened his eyes, snorted a bit, lifted his head and rolled over on his stomach. That was all we needed to see. The farmer gave my friend a wad of cash and said, "That beauty is gonna be walkin' funny fer a while."

On the way back to town, my friend said, "You know, Ron, if you've never tried deep-fried testicles, you don't know what you're missing. The farmer wasn't kidding when he said there're a delicacy. Some folks call them Rocky Mountain oysters."

I wasn't quite that adventurous.

Epilogue:

At the time, I was a chairperson of our local Elks Club (BPOE 1052) and every year in the fall we'd put on a wild-game feed for the members and their families. All the food from their hunting trips was donated to the feed. Club officers did all the cooking and serving and we prepared everything, from big and small game to fish and fowl. There was one particularly unusual item on the menu every year; however, it had a limited appeal.

Our town had another veterinarian, in addition to my friend, whom I also helped out occasionally and who also had an active country practice. Every year for the wild-game feed, he'd bring a large jar of preserved testicles into the kitchen from all the farm-animal castrations he'd done that year saying, "Here you go, boys. Have some nuts!" A couple of the old-timers had a recipe for them that involved seasoned batter and deep-frying. After they were cooked, the veterinarian would bring them around to the tables, offering them to guests as a delicacy from the Rocky Mountains. Most of the folks knew what they were and declined, but occasionally someone who didn't would try one or two and usually said they were delicious. That is, until they found out what they'd eaten.

With a few misgivings, I tried some too. I must admit, there were tasty.

Every year in our little town, the two local veterinarians—my good friend and the other fellow I occasionally helped out—would put on a rabies clinic. This was free for any town resident with small animals. It was advertised well ahead of time so that when the day arrived a lot of folks showed up with their pets and the lines were long. My friend's wife and I were his assistants; she would handle the paperwork and tags for each animal and I'd load syringes with rabies vaccine for him. It was a lot of fun because it was early summer and held in a downtown parking lot on the lakefront. Along with all the people and their pets, plenty of onlookers would show up. It was quite a social event.

Dogs and cats were vaccinated along with bunnies, a few ferrets and even a de-scented baby skunk once. My favorite person in line on one particular day was a sweet little four-year-old farm girl with a cardboard box in her arms. She was the picture of a Scandinavian princess—in blue jeans, cowboy boots, pretty ruffled white blouse and an embroidered jean jacket. Her eyes were blue and her blonde hair fixed with a bright-red bow. She put the box on the table, and my friend said, "Good morning, sweetie. What do you have in the box?"

She told him, "That's my pet kitty, doctor, but he only really likes me and nobody else. And he's kinda mean to strangers, so you hafta be real careful when you reach in there."

My friend said, "Don't worry, honey. I will."

With that, he casually opened the box and reached in. Right away I heard some loud hissing, growling and snarling noises and my friend quickly pulled back a bloodied, scratched-up hand. He wiped it off, looked at the little girl and said, "You're right, honey. That's one mean kitty." He told the little girl that we'd put a towel over the kitty so he couldn't bite anybody, and his assistant would hold him still. Then we'd pull the towel back just far enough to give the kitty his rabies shot, and we'd be all done.

She smiled and said, "Okay, doctor, but be careful." We got the cat "mummied" in the towel, gave him his rabies shot and shut the box. The little girl thanked us and said, "You better see a doctor about your hand."

The life of a small-town veterinarian is the best!

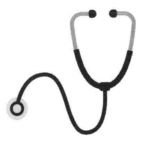

96. Over and Back

Every hospital I worked in had volunteer auxiliary staff. Usually they were retired folks who handled many of the functions of daily hospital routine. They ran the gift shop, manned the information desks, helped out in the waiting rooms and distributed mail to patients, etc.

The surgical waiting room is where family members and friends typically wait to speak to the surgeon after their loved one's operation.

In the late '80s, while working with a mixed group of CRNAs and anesthesiologists at a small hospital in Florida, I got to know Leslie quite well. She was an elderly lady who volunteered at the surgical waiting room desk most days. She was from Australia, had quite an intellect and had a wonderful sense of humor. We became good friends and occasionally would have lunch together in the cafeteria.

For a few months every time I'd pass by the waiting room and peek in there would be somebody different at the desk. Finally, I asked one of the auxiliary ladies where Leslie was. She said, "Oh, you haven't heard? Leslie had a heart attack two months ago. It was a bad one too. They even had to resuscitate her, shock her and everything. Thank Heaven she survived, and now she's home recuperating." I felt bad about that and resigned myself to the fact that her volunteering days were likely over and I'd never see her again.

Quite a while later on my way to lunch, as I passed by the surgical waiting room—lo and behold—there was Leslie back at the desk. We were so glad to see each other that we shared a big hug and I asked her to tell me all about what had happened. She said that she had been at home, not far away from the hospital, when she experienced some severe chest pain. She lived in an assisted living facility so she had her next-door neighbor immediately take her to the ER. When she got there they put oxygen on her and hooked her up to the EKG monitor, and that's the last thing she remembered before waking up in the cardiac ICU later that evening with a very sore chest. The doctor told her that she'd had a heart attack, which caused some bizarre cardiac rhythms, and they had to do CPR on her to overcome them. They even shocked her to cardiovert them back to normal sinus rhythm. She said, "My chest is still very tender from it too."

There was only one other person in the waiting room, so we went over to a corner couch to talk for a while. She told me all about her stay in the cardiac ICU, the medications she was taking now, etc. At one point I said, "Leslie, you and I have been friends for a long time. Could I ask you a personal question, please?"

She said, "Of course."

I said, "I've been in the anesthesia for a long time my dear, and have been in on many codes like yours. Also, sometimes during these events—and after we've successfully resuscitated a person—they wake up so peacefully. One man even described his near-death experience to me in detail. I have to ask: Did you have an 'over and back' experience during the time they were working on you?"

That surprised her, and she looked around to make sure nobody was close by. Then she leaned close to me and said in low tones, "Oh, Ron. Yes, I did and it was wonderful! I was lying on the cart in the ER talking to the doctor, and all of a sudden there was a big, brilliant bright light right in front of me. I floated toward it and as I passed through, I saw the most beautiful pastoral countryside with a lake, blooming flowers everywhere, grassy fields, mountains in the distance and a bunch of people not far away walking toward me. As they got closer, I was so overjoyed to see that it was my dear parents and all the rest of my family coming to greet me. I hugged and kissed every one of them and I asked them if I was dead and this was Heaven. My dad assured me that it was, and that it's a wonderful place. He also told me that I could only be there for a short while because it wasn't my time yet and I had to go back. I didn't want to, Ron. I wanted to stay with my people because I've missed them so much. But my sweet mother told me that it wasn't their decision to make and that it wouldn't be many more years until we're all together."

"And all of a sudden, I woke up crying back in the emergency room with the doctor telling me to take a deep breath. When I finally came to my senses, he asked me why I was crying. I didn't want to share the personal experience I'd just had with him, so I told him it was because my chest hurt. He laughed and told me that they worked on me for about a half hour until they finally got my heart straightened out. I had to thank him for doing it but after seeing Heaven, I really wished he hadn't. So, there you have it, Ron. I haven't shared my experience with anyone else except you. And I'm at complete peace now, because all my questions have been answered."

Her story almost overwhelmed me. I had read accounts of other people's "over and back" experiences that were similar but hearing it firsthand in such vivid detail from my good friend gave me goose bumps. Hers was a truly beautiful experience and I told her so. I thanked Leslie profusely, gave her a big hug and then had to get back to the OR for afternoon cases. After that, Leslie and I would wink whenever we saw each other.

I took a position with a different anesthesia group a year later and left that hospital. I never saw Leslie again, but by now I'm sure she's with her family in the beautiful, pastoral countryside.

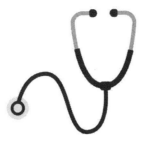

97. Heimlich Maneuver

During lunch one day a bunch of us from the anesthesia department were sitting together in the medical staff dining room with a doctor friend of mine. He was a guy with a great personality who also happened to be the best surgeon I've ever had the pleasure of working with. As we were chatting, the dining room door opened and another member of the medical staff came in followed immediately by a well-dressed young man in a suit and tie. The man in the suit had an agonized look on his face and was clutching at his neck. My surgeon friend leaped out of his chair, ran over to the young man and said in a loud voice, "Can you speak?" The fellow vigorously shook his head no.

My friend quickly got behind him, put his arms around him and gave him a Heimlich maneuver. Nothing came out of the young man's mouth and he was still trying to breathe, so the surgeon performed it on him again. One big cough later, out popped whatever had been obstructing his airway. The young man immediately took a huge breath and stood there for a minute leaning over, hyperventilating and coughing. Finally, when he caught his breath he thanked the surgeon profusely. My friend's only response was, "You won't be thanking me in the morning because I felt a couple of your ribs crack when I was doing that."

The young man left, and my friend returned to the table to finish his lunch. We were all so impressed that we heaped accolades upon him. When I returned to the OR, my hero surgeon friend was already working but hadn't told anybody what had just happened in the lunchroom so I took it upon myself to tell everybody.

What a selfless act.

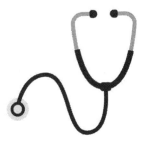

98. My Old Chief CRNA

When I was in anesthesia school, my favorite hospital of all the five I rotated through was North Memorial in Robbinsdale, Minnesota. All the students liked that rotation too because of the excellent chief CRNA and the wide assortment of specialty cases they did in their OR.

The chief had gone through the same program we were in a number of years earlier and had also been a CRNA in the service. He was an outspoken guy with a wry sense of humor who didn't shrink from being brutally frank when the situation called for it and some of his quips and one-liners were so appropriate and funny. Here are just a few situations where they came into play:

One morning he was on a case with an irascible surgeon who continually complained about everything, including the quality of the anesthetic. The chief finally stood up, looked over the ether screen, which is the U-shaped bar over the patient that holds the drapes separating the surgical field from the anesthesia provider, and said to the surgeon, while pointing to the ether screen, "Do you know what this is, doctor?" The surgeon looked at it and said, "Sure, that's the ether screen." The chief said, "No, it's the blood-brain barrier—you're the blood, and I'm the brain." He sat down and the surgeon finished the case without another word.

Anesthesia providers are always aware of the level and quality of a surgical patient's anesthetic while they're asleep. That and patient safety are the main focus of our profession. Common jargon in the OR when referring to levels of anesthetic depth is "light," for when they've just been put to sleep, and "deep," referring to their state during the middle of a procedure. Surgeons pick up on these terms and sometimes make reference to them during the case. The chief was on a case one morning with a whiney surgeon and in the middle of it the surgeon muttered about the patient being a little "light." The chief, knowing full well that the patient was deeply anesthetized, made him repeat it and then said, "Just a minute, doctor, and I'll darken him for you." Not another word was said after that.

One day, during a procedure, a circulating nurse was constantly telling the chief what the patient needed and when to do certain things relative to the anesthetic. When he'd finally had enough of it he said to her, "Listen, I can do your job. Can you do mine?" She sat down and shut up.

We got word in the OR that two ambulances were coming in with some severely injured people from a car wreck and that they would probably need anesthesia personnel in the ER to help with IVs and handle airway issues. The chief and I got there just after they'd brought in four people and he told me to quickly intubate one of the men on the ambulance stretcher whose face looked pretty blue so I grabbed some airway equipment and ran over to him. He wasn't breathing, so I quickly put a laryngoscope blade in his mouth and looked down his throat for the glottic opening into his trachea.

When I found it, instead of it being very dark, it seemed to be a pale blue. I put the endotracheal tube in right away and when I hooked the AMBU bag to the tube there was a massive air leak coming from under the sheet over the patient. When the nurse who was with me pulled the sheet back, the reason for the leak was obvious. The patient's neck was completely transected and not connected to his body at all—with about a two-inch gap between the two. The pale-blue color I had seen while looking through his glottic opening was light coming through the blue sheet that covered him. Evidently, the ambulance crew just loaded him on the stretcher without being aware of it. The chief's comment was, "Maybe this fellow wouldn't mind if we took his head back to the department and let all the students practice intubating it."

In the middle of the case a surgeon once told him that the patient didn't seem to be bleeding very much, implying that the blood pressure was very low due to deep anesthesia. The chief told him, "Well I know you're in your element, trying to control all the bleeding you cause, so if it will make you happy I could give the patient a big dose of blood thinner. Would that make you more comfortable?" That ended any further conversation.

The anesthesiologists in that department never did cases; they practiced supervisory anesthesia. They would come to our room when we were ready to start a case, inject drugs to put the patient to sleep and leave. The CRNA would do the rest of the case alone. The chief was doing a case one morning and got called to an important meeting with the hospital administrator. It was a busy day and no other CRNA was available to relieve him so he called for the chief anesthesiologist (MDA) to come in the room. When he arrived, the chief gave him report and went off to his meeting. After a half hour he was back, got the report from the MDA and took over the case. When the MDA had left the room, the surgeon turned to the chief and said, "Damn, that was the worst half hour of a case I've ever had to deal with. Thank Heaven you're back."

I was doing an abdominal aortic aneurysm repair case one morning. These were complicated major surgery cases on sick patients that often required intraoperative blood transfusions. The surgeon, although competent, didn't have a very pleasant personality and usually took a long time to do these kinds of cases. At times during the case, my patient had been unstable requiring blood transfusions and many drugs to keep him safe. Our anesthesia records were in two parts with carbon paper in between. One copy went to the patient's chart and the other to the anesthesia billing office. My record that day, because of the patient's instability, had a lot of notations on it, even writing in the margins.

At noon, the chief came in to relieve me for lunch. When I came back, the case was almost over and the surgeon was starting to close. When I looked at my anesthesia record, in the space where the type of surgical procedure was normally entered, the chief had written in big block letters, "HOMICIDE." I was rattled! I couldn't turn in a record with that written on it. That meant I would have to recopy the whole record over again after the operation—and quickly, because there were cases to follow in my room and turnover times were short. When we got to the recovery room, I yelled for another anesthesia record, gave report to the nurse and started copying furiously. I was just finishing up when they called me for the next case. Fortunately, we had an excellent anesthesia technician in the department and she had my room all set up for me.

When the day finished, I saw the chief in the locker room and started to let him know what I thought of his prank. Before I finished he said, "Now you learned that you're supposed to check everything during a case, even the chart."

He was, without a doubt, the best CRNA I ever had the good fortune to work with. He was a skilled practitioner and had excellent leadership and teaching skills. He ran an anesthesia department that covered ten operating rooms, two dental suites and obstetrics, and was respected by everybody. And had a soft heart.

Of all the CRNAs I worked with during my schooling, he was without a doubt the best. His influence remained the driving force behind all my critical thinking and practice techniques and I am forever indebted to him for my successful career.

We still keep in touch.

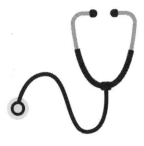

99. HIV Epidural

In 1988 the AIDS/HIV epidemic was a significant concern to all healthcare workers. Occasionally, we'd have a patient needing surgery who was infected and the precautions by the OR personnel involved in the care of that person were extreme. Anesthesia providers were especially vulnerable to the infection by virtue of being close to the patient's bodily fluids while starting IVs, intubating their airway and suctioning secretions.

One afternoon I was called to obstetrics for a labor epidural and when I arrived, the nurse attending the patient told me to be very careful because the patient had AIDS. That made me nervous, to say the least, because to perform the epidural I would be handling several needles and injecting her back. Once, during an epidural, a lady jumped as I infiltrated her back with lidocaine at the epidural site and it made my syringe jerk sideways sticking me in the finger with the needle. That incident was still fresh in my mind as I prepared to meet the woman.

She was a pleasant young woman who was laboring with her first pregnancy. After I introduced myself, she was quite candid and emotional telling me that she got AIDS from unprotected sex with a new boyfriend. She also said that she knew she was going to die a horrible death because of it, but just wanted to see her baby before that happened and that she was going to put the baby up for adoption. Then she burst into tears. It was probably the most gut-wrenching interview I've ever had with a patient. She didn't have anybody with her, and I didn't ask why.

An OB nurse came to help me with the epidural and we both put on gowns, gloves (I double-gloved), masks and protective glasses. She sat the lady up and I put in her epidural without any problems, being extremely careful whenever I had a needle or syringe in my hands. When we were finished, and the lady was comfortable, she thanked us profusely and started to sob again. The nurse started to cry too and I had to leave the room to collect myself and do my charting out in the hallway. When I saw her nurse later I asked her to please mention the poor woman's emotional state to her doctor and get her some professional help.

That was at a time when AIDS/HIV was scarier than the coronavirus is today because in those days HIV/AIDS was almost a certain death, and the coronavirus mortality these days is much less than that. Since then, and due to many years of dedicated research, a lot of different drugs have been developed that are effectively available to treat the HIV virus and, if taken correctly, it's possible for infected individuals to have a relatively normal lifespan.

I often wonder what happened to that young woman.

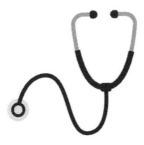

100. Bleeding Tonsil

In the 1970s tonsillectomies on young children were much more common than they are now and generally speaking the little people were not very happy about having it done. At our small hospital in northern Minnesota I usually needed several people to help me get them to sleep and start their IVs because very few of the children were cooperative and once they left the arms of their mom they often got hysterical. They usually had to be held down, kicking and screaming, on the OR table by a couple of nurses while I did an inhalation induction of anesthesia. Once the child was asleep, a circulator would start their IV, I'd intubate them and the case would get underway.

Their emergence from anesthesia was a critical time because there was always a little blood in their throat, the tonsil beds (fossae) would be raw, and I needed them to be awake enough to have their airway reflexes intact before I removed the endotracheal tube. Usually they woke up coughing, crying and screaming, and I worried that it might start some bleeding. Fortunately, that rarely happened. Occasionally, though, the tonsil fossae could bleed within the first week postoperatively for many reasons. When this happened, the child would usually bleed (mostly ooze) in their throat, spit some blood out of their mouth and swallow a good deal of it, which made the family very upset and worried when they brought them into the ER.

These cases are always a real anesthetic challenge because of a full stomach, blood in the airway and a very frightened child. Plus, they can also be somewhat dehydrated from blood loss. To protect their airway, a rapid sequence induction of anesthesia is essential.

One morning, my first case of the day was a tonsillectomy on a cute little five-year-old girl. When I went to see the family preoperatively, they were a very happy bunch. She had her teddy bear with her and was with her mom and dad. After introducing myself, I asked her if she was glad to be getting rid of those "nasty" old tonsils and she said, "Yes sir I am. And my teacher said I could bring them to school for show and tell."

What a clever ruse to get her to look forward to a tonsillectomy. I asked her if she wouldn't mind blowing up a balloon to go to sleep today, and her face lit up because she said it was one of her favorite things to do. I told her we'd take good care of her and as I reached over to pat her on the head, she leaned forward and gave me a big hug. It's not very often that a five-year-old is that well-adjusted and cooperative.

The case went very well and, although she woke up crying, she was fine as soon as she saw her mom. She went home later that day.

The following Saturday morning I was called to the hospital for a bleeding tonsil. I knew immediately who the patient was because the cute little girl was the only tonsillectomy case we'd had that week. When I arrived, the frightened family was in the ER and the little patient was whimpering and sitting on her mom's lap. Her lips had dried blood on them and every so often her mom would have her spit into a hanky. She recognized me right away and managed a weak smile. I told her that we'd get her all fixed up but asked if she'd mind a little "mosquito" bite in the hand this time instead of blowing up the balloon. She said, "Okay." That was a relief because it meant we wouldn't have to wrestle with her to get an IV started.

The OR team was there and after everything was set up we let the little girl's mother carry her, and her teddy bear, into the OR suite where she stayed with her in the recovery room while I got her IV started. Once that was done, Mom left and we brought the girl into the OR. I let her breathe some oxygen, the circulator put a little pressure on her neck right below the Adam's apple and I injected Pentothal and muscle relaxant into her IV so I could quickly intubate her. Once she was asleep, the surgeon found the area in one of her tonsil fossae that was oozing and cauterized it. I had him slip a gastric tube into her stomach to empty out whatever blood she might have swallowed. The case was over in about fifteen minutes.

She woke up crying, so we brought Mom in which made her smile. I had given her 150 ccs of normal saline during surgery to catch her up on her fluids and she looked good. By the time she was wide awake, she was smiling again. She had her teddy bear, so I got a surgical mask and put it on teddy and gave her one too. I told her to take it with her, along with her tonsils, for show and tell.

We kept her a few more hours and let her go home.

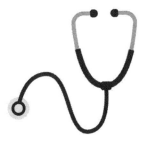

101. Deer Hunting Gunshot Injuries

Deer hunting season in Minnesota is almost a state holiday and our little northern town was surrounded by many square miles of lakes and woods, providing an excellent environment for deer. The rifle season usually opens the second week of November and during that time the woods are full of hunters—lots of them from Minneapolis. Once the season is open, and the shooting starts, deer get the jitters and are on the move day and night which can make driving on country roads dangerous. One could jump out in front of your vehicle without warning. If a vehicle hits a deer and it isn't smashed up badly, the driver can call the DNR (Department of Natural Resources) to report it and then take the carcass home or to a locker plant to be cut and wrapped for personal consumption.

Deer season also brought a lot of business to our little hospital. We'd get everything from heart attacks on overweight hunters trying to drag a two hundred-pound buck a mile out of the woods, broken bones from tree-related falls, cut tendons from a sharp knife field dressing the deer, to a variety of accidental gunshot wounds.

My favorite idiotic gunshot wound case involved a hunter who came in shortly after sunrise on opening day. He had a tree stand twenty-five feet up in a large pine tree that he couldn't climb to while holding his rifle so he tied a rope around it, climbed up to the stand and then pulled the rifle up after him. The only problem was that he didn't bother to unload the rifle first, didn't check to see that the safety was on and, worst of all, he tied the pull-up rope to the muzzle of the rifle. He got into his stand and as he was pulling his rifle up, the trigger caught on a branch discharging a round of 30-06 ammo up through his foot and leg and out his hip. It was an expanding round too, so as it traversed his leg it tore up all the soft tissue and fractured a lot of bones. Fortunately, it went up the side of his leg and didn't get the femoral artery or he never would have made it out of the woods alive. He then fell out of the tree and broke his shoulder when he hit the ground. Lucky he didn't break his neck. A friend heard him screaming and was nearby to help him and bring him to the hospital. All we could do was x-ray him, explore his leg for bleeding, clean his wounds and call for the plane from Minneapolis to come get him.

Another crazy shooting incident occurred when two friends from out of town went to the same spot they'd hunted in for years. It was on the top of two hills on either side of a swale. They were directly across from one another on the hilltops and about one hundred yards apart, each sitting in a tree stand ten feet off the ground. Deer evidently used a trail down in the swale so the mighty hunters didn't mind being in each other's possible line of fire. Evidently, a big buck came down the trail and one of the hunters took a shot at it and missed. The scared deer, instead of running down the trail, ran up the hill opposite of the hunter who shot at it. Having missed his first shot, and excited to see such a big deer, the guy took aim again. As he pulled the trigger, the deer moved right into the line of fire of his friend. He missed the deer again and instead shot his buddy out of the tree with a 30-30 slug.

Fortunately, the guy had a thick hunting jacket on and the bullet hit him in the soft tissue just under his left rib cage leaving a deep flesh wound. The force of the slug's impact was enough to knock him out of the tree and he broke his arm when he hit the ground. He was very lucky. We just cleaned up his flesh wound, set his arm, and sent him on his way. His parting words were, "Well, now I can just sit in camp and drink for the rest of the week."

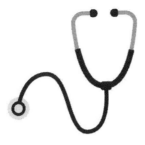

102. Engine Block

Another visiting deer hunter went out to his favorite spot ten miles north of town and drove his four-wheel-drive truck down an old logging road two miles back into the woods to a little grassy meadow. He left his pickup, loaded his rifle and walked about fifty yards across the clearing when a spooked deer ran between him and the truck right behind him. He turned around and shot, missing the deer but putting the slug of a .300 magnum through the pickup's engine block. It was a long walk back to the sparsely traveled main road and a long time before he got a ride to town.

Pretty expensive hunting trip…

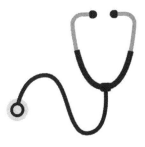

103. The '63 Ford Pickup

I got called to the hospital late one night in the '70s during deer season for a ruptured spleen case on a hunter who had fallen out of a tree. Because I was in a hurry, I took my old '63 Ford pickup that was parked in the turnaround of my yard. Ruptured spleens cause major bleeding, so when I got to the main road from my driveway I stepped on it. A half mile down the road I saw movement out of the corner of my eye and in a flash a deer ran right in front of the truck. I hit it dead center at about 65 mph.

I saw the deer fly off into the ditch but the headlights were still working and my old Ford, built like a Sherman tank, was running fine so I had to keep going. I got to the hospital and did the case, saving a patient who had lost a lot of blood, and went to inspect the front of my truck with a flashlight. It was covered with hair and blood.

I remembered the spot where I hit the deer, so on my way home I stopped and went looking for it. It took me a while and when I finally did find the poor thing, it was about fifty feet off the road. There wasn't much left. The old Ford was so sturdy and I had been going so fast that the deer died instantly.

Glad it didn't suffer.

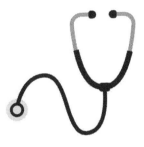

104. Foreign Bodies

On a wintery Sunday morning in northern Minnesota, I was notified that I needed to come to the hospital for a child who had swallowed a penny. When I arrived in the ER, the patient, a cute little three-year-old curly-haired boy, was sitting on his mother's lap and not in any particular distress. His mother explained that she had been getting ready for church and had her purse out, letting her little boy play with three pennies while she got ready. When she was all set to go she saw only two pennies on the table. She asked her son where the other penny was and he pointed to his mouth. She looked in there but didn't see a trace of the penny. He wasn't having any trouble breathing so she was pretty sure it wasn't in his airway. She was worried that it might be caught in his esophagus though. Fortunately, he had eaten a light breakfast very early that morning and it was almost noon now so I wasn't extremely concerned about a full stomach.

We sent the little boy to X-Ray to see where the penny was. When the film came back it showed the penny at the very upper end of his esophagus. I consulted with the surgeon on call and we decided that we might be able to see it on a throat exam after he was asleep.

Mom brought the child to the surgery, and we put a surgical gown on her so she could go into the OR and be with him and he'd be cooperative while I gave him a little inhalation anesthetic. She held him sitting up, and I blew anesthetic vapors across his face until he started getting woozy. Then she laid him down and I was able to put the mask on his face and anesthetize him. Her only comment was, "That stuff smells sickeningly sweet." Then she left and went out to the waiting room.

After he was deeply anesthetized and breathing spontaneously, I carefully put a pediatric laryngoscope blade into his mouth and slid it down to the base of his tongue. I could see the tip of the penny just barely protruding from the top of his esophagus. With a special instrument, called a Magill forceps, I carefully grabbed the penny and pulled it out. That was a stroke of luck; if it had been down further the procedure would've been much more complicated.

The whole case took about fifteen minutes and the little boy woke up without a whimper so we returned him to his smiling mother's arms. I told her to save the penny and keep it for good luck.

My partner and I became quite adept at throat exams in the '70s and '80s, especially in the summer, since many vacationers came to our area resorts to fish for walleyes. After catching a full stringer, all those fish would need to be cleaned for dinner and very few of them knew how to do a professional job of it. Consequently, a few small bones often remained in the fillets. After some celebratory drinks over the day's catch, a fish fry would often commence among the happy vacationers and about once or twice a week a fisherman would come to the ER in the evening complaining of a fishbone caught in his throat.

Because they almost always had been drinking and had food in their stomachs, we didn't put them to sleep to examine their throats. Instead, we'd spray their mouth and throats with an atomizer of topical lidocaine to make them numb and then do a throat exam with our laryngoscope. About 90 percent of the time we couldn't find anything. Usually there would only be a small redness in one of their tonsil fossae from the irritation a fishbone had made while they were swallowing it and which made them feel like something was there. Occasionally, if a small bone *was* stuck, we could grab it with the Magill forceps.

It kept us busy. Unfortunately though, most of this type of work occurred during the evenings or middle of the night.

Another thing fishermen kept the ER staff busy with was removing fishhooks from various parts of their anatomy. My partner and I didn't usually have to be involved, since the hook could be pushed through soft tissue until the barb was sticking out, whereupon it would be cut off and the hook pulled back and out.

The ER had a life-sized diagram of a fisherman hanging on the wall and every time they took a hook out of somebody they'd hook one on the diagram in a corresponding spot. By the end of the summer the diagram had so many hooks in it they were just about all you could see.

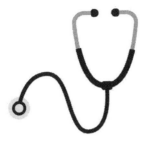

105. Car Wreck

At 2 a.m. on a below-zero night in January 1973, I was called to the hospital for a man badly injured in a car/grain truck accident a mile west of town. I hurried into the hospital and arrived just as the ambulance was pulling up to the ER. The highway patrol trooper told me that our patient was a passenger in a car driving at a high rate of speed out on the highway and had run into the back end of a moving, loaded grain truck. The car slid completely under the truck, killing the other five people in the car. Our patient was the only survivor; they found him lying on the floor of the back seat, which was probably what saved him.

The man was marginally conscious. When we got him on an ER cart I started two large bore IVs, with warm normal saline, in each arm and drew blood for lab work and a type and crossmatch. His vital signs were low but stable and he was extremely cold from the below-zero weather while he had been lying in the car waiting to be extracted but he was breathing well so we put an oxygen mask on him. Both of his legs were laying at obtuse angles between his hips and knees, and one foot looked crunched. His face had multiple lacerations—probably from flying glass—and a sizable hematoma was on the top of his head, which we were concerned might be hiding a fractured skull underneath it. The nurses put a few warm blankets on him after they got his bloody clothes off, and I went to get my room ready for the case.

When we got the fellow on the OR table and I anesthetized him right away without a problem and we called X-Ray to come see how bad his fractures were. He had bilateral, severely fractured femurs and many fractures in one foot, but his chest and arms were okay. The surgeon said, "He's damn lucky to have survived, let alone not gotten a broken neck out of this wreck."

For the next four hours we did surgery on his fractured femurs, sutured up his many facial lacerations, and casted his foot. I took him to the ICU to wake up as the sun was coming up. He was breathing on his own at that point with the endotracheal tube still in place and after about an hour he woke up enough for me to remove it.

He had a neurological workup and it turned out that he had a small fracture in his skull under that hematoma. He was in the hospital for a long time and after discharge had an even longer rehab.

It was a somber atmosphere in the OR that night because one of the ladies killed in the terrible crash had been a good friend of ours. She was a pretty, young gal who had worked in central supply at the hospital.

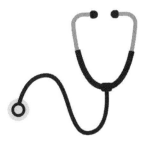

106. Demerol Anesthesia

A normal IV dose of Demerol to control postoperative pain in the recovery room is 5 to 25 mg depending upon the severity. Its half-life is between two and five hours and incremental doses are administered to the patient per the recovery room nurse's or attending anesthesia personnel's judgment. Demerol is not used in the recovery room much anymore because of its propensity to cause nausea—and also because there are better drugs available now.

When I was a senior anesthesia student in the late '60s, one of the large metropolitan hospitals I rotated through had an unusual non-mainstream technique of administering general anesthesia to all their adult patients. The chief anesthesiologist had developed it, and it was mandated by him for all those cases. Basically, his protocol was a deep Demerol narcosis anesthetic, which stayed with the patient for many hours postoperatively.

After the induction of anesthesia, with pentothal and a muscle relaxant, the patient was intubated. The formula for anesthetic maintenance after induction was 20 milligrams of Demerol IV every twenty minutes for the duration of the case, along with light inhalation anesthetic vapors. If it happened to be a big case that took many hours, the total dose of Demerol to the patient could amount to a quite few hundred milligrams. All this was, of course, relative to the patient's vital signs and ability to handle that regimen, but all adults received whatever doses of Demerol they could tolerate.

Also, part of the chief's mandate was that no muscle relaxants, which render the patient unable to breathe without support and cause striated muscle to become flaccid to facilitate surgical exposure, could be reversed at the end of the procedure. Instead, the muscle relaxant had to be allowed to be metabolized or "worn off" in the recovery room for however long that might take. As you can imagine, a patient's stay in the recovery room could last a very long time.

When a surgical case was finished, and the patient had received the perfunctory dose of Demerol and still had unmetabolized muscle relaxant affecting their ability to breathe spontaneously, the CRNA would call into the recovery room and announce, "I'm bringing a patient with a tube." When the recovery room responded that there was a slot open, we'd move the patient to a cart, give them a few big breaths of pure oxygen, disconnect the anesthesia machine breathing hoses from their endotracheal tube and run like hell to the recovery room. Upon our arrival, a nurse would always be standing ready for the patient with a positive pressure breathing valve apparatus attached to an oxygen line and operated by a push button in her hand. She would attach that to their endotracheal tube and ventilate the patient at about twelve breaths per minute until the muscle relaxant and respiratory depressant effects of the Demerol wore off.

Depending on the dosages of those two drugs that the patient had received during surgery, it could take hours before they were out of their system and frequently they woke up nauseated. While I was there, one patient who'd had a long operation that finished in the late afternoon ended up in the recovery room all night with a nurse ventilating him by hand until the drugs wore off. Sometimes afterward, they would completely lose a day because of the associated retrograde amnesia due to the long-term effects of Demerol.

This approach to general anesthesia was not practiced anywhere else in the hospitals associated with our anesthesia program and has long since been discarded. If we used Demerol at all during surgery at other places back then, it was only as a small supplemental dose once or twice during a big case in which the patient was receiving a large amount of surgical stimulation. And all muscle relaxants, with few exceptions, were reversed with antagonist drugs at the end of the case. An ideal emergence from anesthesia is to have the patient lightly sedated, relatively pain-free, arousable, breathing spontaneously, and well-oriented.

As unique as this Demerol technique was, it was excellent training for all of us. Narcotics are an integral part of today's practice of anesthesia and the modern ones have evolved into much more potent drugs that have a predictable duration with fewer side effects.

We used to joke amongst ourselves about giving a pound of Demerol to our patients every day.

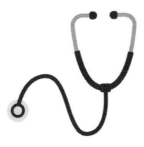

107. Old Soldier Hip Fracture

In the mid-'70s, repair of some hip fractures required a replacement ball prosthesis to fit into the socket of the patient's acetabulum. Usually these patients were elderly and in a marginal to poor state of health, thus making it imperative to fix their hips quickly so they wouldn't have to lay inactive in a hospital bed for very long which could lead to pneumonia.

I was called to the hospital one Saturday afternoon for a hip fracture case on an eighty-five-year-old man. His daughter was with him and told me that he had a bit of dementia and lived mostly in the past. The old fellow had a cute personality and told me that he had been an infantryman in the Second World War. "…and I ran up Mt. Suribachi with the boys to beat back them Japs." His lab work was fine, but he wasn't very healthy because of COPD and a history of heart disease. The anesthetic of choice in those days for old folks needing hip surgery was spinal anesthesia.

We brought the old guy to the OR and, with the circulating nurse's help, I put in a spinal anesthetic then we positioned him on his side. Because of his health problems I didn't dare sedate him much, only giving him very small incremental doses of pentothal periodically. The surgery got underway and he was comfortable. He would snooze for a while after a dose of pentothal, wake up and fidget a bit, look around, and ask me questions like, "What the hell kind of a barracks is this?" When he heard the surgeon tapping a reamer down the shaft of his femur, he snapped out, "What in the hell is that? Are we under attack again? Damn. Call in the artillery!"

The funniest of all was when he woke up and noticed the surgeon reach up—with a bloody glove—to grasp the sterile overhead light handle and adjust

289

it. In a loud voice the old soldier said, "What'cha got on your hands there, boy? Is that blood? Damn, you better find yourself a medic and get the hell over to a field tent real quick. It looks pretty bad." That made us all laugh.

The surgery went well, and after an hour we had our soldier over to the ICU for recovery. I told the nurses there to brush up on their World War II history because their patient was still fighting a few of those battles.

A few months later I saw him downtown with his daughter and as I walked by I saluted him and said, "Good morning, Colonel." He gave me a big smile and saluted back.

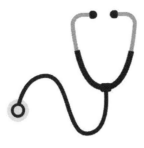

108. The Art Gallery

Mid-morning, I was notified that an emergency carotid endarterectomy case was coming into my room. This is a very demanding case, as I've described earlier, but this one was more critical than most because the patient was an elderly man in ICU recovering from a recent serious heart attack.

I went to see him in ICU and was impressed by how sick he appeared. His lab work was marginal, he had multiple IV pumps running in each arm with potent medications in them, an arterial line in his wrist, an oxygen mask on his face and his cardiac monitor tracing was slightly irregular, consistent with major heart damage. His anxious wife told me that he was also suffering from significant dementia, but since this carotid issue happened it had become worse. She also said that the doctor had told her if he didn't have this operation, he'd be a total vegetable in no time. I reassured her that the surgeon was excellent and even though her husband was critically ill, we'd do our best to make him better.

She was frightened, and I was concerned that we might have some real problems with him during surgery.

With a lot of help, we got the old fellow to the OR and on the table. It took a while to sort out all his lines and transfer them to my anesthesia monitors, but once that was done my attending anesthesiologist and I cautiously anesthetized him. He tolerated the induction of anesthesia marginally well, and soon the surgery was underway. His vital signs were extremely labile during the case and I was constantly adjusting my anesthetic gasses and his IV pump medications to keep them marginally stable. The surgery went well and ended relatively quickly. At the end of the case I decided not to remove his endotracheal tube, instead taking him back to ICU and placing him on a ventilator for safety. His wife was there when we arrived. After I got all his monitors and IV lines transferred, I had a discussion with her about why he would be on the ventilator for a while.

The guy was so critically ill and unstable that I was sure he wouldn't live much longer and discussed that with my attending anesthesiologist when I got back to the department. We were both thankful he didn't have a cardiac arrest on the OR table.

About a year later, my wife and I were in downtown St. Petersburg on a Saturday afternoon and stopped at a small art gallery gift shop. The owner came over to see if she could help us find something and to my surprise, it was the wife of the sick old fellow from the carotid case. I introduced myself as the person who had put her husband to sleep for surgery a year before and I fully expected her to tell me that he didn't survive the ordeal but instead she said, "Go say hi to him. He's sitting behind the counter over there. He won't remember you because he has some pretty significant dementia, but he's very pleasant." I went over and had a little conversation with my old patient and she was right; he had no idea who I was and didn't recall a thing about ever being in the hospital.

Before we left I couldn't help but tell her how glad I was that he had survived, because I truly never thought he would. She agreed and hugged me.

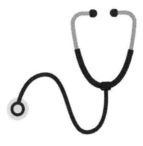

109. Alcohol Infusion

In the early '70s, one of the treatments for impending DTs in our little North Country hospital was to give the patient an IV infusion of 5 percent alcohol. Alcoholism wasn't the main reason for their admission usually, but an alcoholic might be hospitalized for a medical condition or for some essential surgical procedure and even a few days of abstinence could trigger an episode of DTs.

An old fellow, a confirmed drinker, had been an inpatient for about a week and because of his debilitated condition was being treated medically for stomach ulcers. As a precaution his doctor had ordered an IV alcohol infusion to be started on him. Over the course of his stay he hadn't responded well to treatment which, in hospital jargon, was referred to as having the "dwindles." No amount of treatment or nourishment seemed to have much of a positive therapeutic effect on him and his doctor was stumped.

One day his wife paid him a visit and was alarmed at the sad state he was in and instead of consulting with anyone, she opened up the IV drip and emptied the whole bottle, 1000cc's of 5% alcohol, into him in a matter of minutes. The old man immediately brightened up, called for something to eat and was discharged the next day.

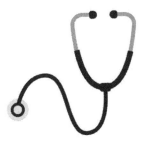

110. Three Stories Before My Shift at the Hospital

My wife and I moved to the Tampa Bay area of Florida in 1987. I took a position with a mixed group of anesthesiologists and CRNAs at a small hospital and she opened a small restaurant with a Minnesota theme and recipes. She introduced wild rice bread to the area, which became so popular that within eight years she had opened five locations. If I worked an afternoon shift at the hospital I'd go to one of the cafes in the morning to help out. I usually worked the register—the easiest task for me considering my limited food-prep skills—and also it gave me a chance to talk to the customers.

Cars registered in Florida only need a rear license plate. Consequently, many folks opted to have some kind of personalized plate on the front end.

One morning I was helping out at one of her restaurants where the cash register was in a direct line of sight with the glass entry door. A car pulled up just outside the door that had a decorative front plate on it that read, "Mary" in beautifully scripted artwork. A well-dressed lady in a business suit got out and came in. When she got to the register, I said, "Hi, Mary."

She looked over her glasses, clearly surprised, and asked, "Have we met?"

I jokingly said, "Yes, we have. Don't you remember? It was at the Fine Arts Center for a fundraiser about a month ago."

She smiled and said, "Oh, yes. Now I remember. How are you?" She extended her hand to shake mine.

I said, "Mary, hold it just a minute. Look out the door at the front plate on your car."

She turned, saw it and then said, "Oh, my god. I'm so embarrassed."

I couldn't stifle a big laugh and told her, "Please, don't be. I just couldn't pass an opportunity like that up. Let me buy you lunch for being such a good sport."

She laughed too. I bought her lunch and she was a good customer from then on.

The schedule finished up early one day while I was working the morning shift at the hospital, so I went to my wife's restaurant a little before closing to talk to the manager and pick up the day's receipts. As we were discussing things in the back room, I thought I heard the door open. I turned around to see who it was and found a very skinny old man standing right behind me. I said, "Hi. How're you?"

"Just fine," he said.

I said, "My name's Ron. What's yours?"

"Andy," he replied.

"How about a bottle of water, Andy?" I asked.

He nodded and said, "That'd be good."

I asked him where he was from and he told me Philadelphia. He obviously had a bit of dementia and I wondered what he was doing wandering around all by himself. I happened to glance past him out the window and saw a couple of middle-aged ladies running frantically all over the parking lot. I said, "Come on over here with me Andy, I want you to see something." I took him by the hand, led him out the front door and yelled, "Girls, is this who you're looking for?"

They let out a screech, ran over to us and one of them asked, "Where on earth did you find him?"

I told them he had just wandered into the shop a few minutes earlier. I learned that they were his daughters and had left him sleeping in the back seat of the car with the doors locked. One back window had been left halfway down while they went into the dry cleaners next door. They showed me that the doors were still locked, so he must've crawled out through that half-open window.

I asked her if he really was from Philly, and she said, "Yeah, seventy years ago. Now he's an eighty-six-year-old five-year-old."

I laughed and said, "Well, you better get him home pretty quick, ladies, because I gave him a bottle of water."

"*Oh, Lord!*" the one daughter exclaimed, and they loaded him into the car and drove off.

I hoped they made it home (and to a bathroom) in time.

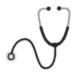

When my wife's restaurant in downtown St. Petersburg, Florida was new and had only been open for about a year it was a very busy place. It had a dining room for indoor eating and also operated a big takeout and delivery lunch catering business. I didn't know any of the staff except the manager, so when I was there in the mornings occasionally to help out I was either assigned some menial task or I just talked to the customers.

One particularly busy morning, everybody—including the manager—was scurrying about getting huge early catering orders ready and nobody was available to run the cash register. I had done it a couple of times in my wife's other smaller restaurants, so she assigned me that job until everyone got caught up. I was familiar with the menu but not all the prices of each item. When a customer gave me their order, I had to take a minute or two to look them up and figure out their bill.

As it got closer to the lunch hour, walk-in traffic got a lot heavier. Due to my lack of speed figuring out each customer's ticket the line at the register got longer and longer, until it stretched out the door and into the street. When the manager saw that, she rushed over and said, "There's a big lunch order getting ready for one of the drivers to deliver and they need thirty cups of ice to go with it. Why don't you go fill the cups for that order and I'll knock this line out in a couple of minutes." I was happy to do that rather than hold up all those hungry people.

I went to the back of the shop and started filling cups with ice. One of the salad prep ladies, who didn't know me, came over as I was doing it and said in low tones, "She took you off the register, huh?"

I said, "Yes, she did, and I'm glad because that was even more stressful than my other job!"

She looked at me with a warm smile, patted my shoulder, and said, "Oh, you have another job? That's really good. I'm so glad to hear that."

She was concerned for the newly hired old guy who obviously wasn't going to last long.

Evidently, she didn't know that I signed her checks and slept with the owner.

Author's Note

In the last third of my anesthesia career, I developed a deadly blood and immune system cancer called multiple myeloma. Before that I was in excellent physical condition, was working full time and riding my bike about nine miles three times a week. The early symptoms I experienced were extreme bone pain in my ribs and sternum (breast bone) and thoracic spine, which I attributed to exercising, followed by a cold that went on to pneumonia and put me in the hospital.

Once the diagnosis was made by my oncologist, and the pneumonia cured, I had a long summer of outpatient chemotherapy designed to put me into remission for the ultimate goal of having a stem cell transplant. My chiefs of anesthesia couldn't have been more accommodating during that period and I was able to work for a few months doing easy cases until the time for the transplant drew near. I took a leave of absence in early December 2011 and had the stem cell transplant at Moffitt Cancer Hospital in Tampa, Florida on December 16. I went back to work part time in June 2012 and full time in August 2012.

I continue to be in remission and have monthly infusions of an immunotherapy drug, along with some pills, to keep me that way. I have two oncologists and their excellent support staffs watching over me now and I feel good. But I have to admit, after everything that's happened I feel much older. I also developed even more empathy for all patients after going through this experience.

I had always been sensitive to my patients' anxieties in facing whatever medical or surgical problems they had, but after being on the other side of things and dealing with my own awful fears about the outcome and side effects of a stem cell transplant to cure multiple myeloma, I developed a deep compassion for all suffering. I'm active now on a multiple myeloma blog and give advice to people about how to handle their treatment and the many side effects of the disease.

The two episodes that follow are about incidents that happened to me during and around the time of my stem cell ordeal. They affected me deeply and changed a great deal of my perspective about life. I suffered a bit with survivor's guilt afterwards because I had made many friends with multiple myeloma during my chemotherapy sessions and some of them didn't respond well and died.

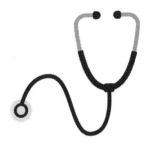

111. Angel's Visit

I developed a cold in May 2011. It lingered for a week or two, and I started on antibiotics. It still got progressively worse to the point that I was having trouble breathing. After the third week of this dyspnea (shortness of breath), Lonni caught me sleeping sitting in an armchair on the sun porch and gave me an ultimatum: either go to the emergency room willingly or she'd call 911. Needless to say, I went willingly.

When I got to the ER my O2 saturation on room air was 82 percent! I had a chest x-ray and blood work that confirmed pneumonia and I was admitted and started on IV antibiotics. The next morning, my doctor said, "The chest/rib pain you're experiencing is much worse than what you get from just coughing from pneumonia so I want to get a CT scan of your chest."

The day after the CT scan, he came into my room with a serious look on his face, shutting the door behind him. He said the CT showed all kinds of lytic fractures (pathologic fractures from invasive cancer) in my ribs and spine, and that I either had a metastatic cancer from somewhere or I had multiple myeloma which is a cancer that affects plasma cells in the body and that I would need a bone marrow biopsy to confirm the diagnosis. I was beyond stunned. I wasn't even a little prepared to hear that and I was all by myself, Lonni hadn't arrived yet.

Hard to describe the disconnect I experienced at that moment. It was as though I was floating in the vapors for a few minutes with my head spinning and a combination of fear and detachment from reality gripping me, feeling totally immobilized and helpless, trying to deal with emotions and anxieties that were extreme.

Lonni arrived about an hour later, and it took quite a while for us to come to grips with the situation. Later that day, I went for a bone marrow biopsy and the diagnosis of multiple myeloma was confirmed. Fortunately, I was a patient in the hospital where I worked, so over the course of the next week my coworkers all came by to bolster my morale. What a great group!

I saw an oncologist that day, who laid out the course of treatment I would have to follow: chemotherapy for the rest of the summer and a stem cell transplant in the fall or winter.

Pneumonia cured, I went home weak as a kitten and had outpatient chemotherapy every week the rest of the summer. In October 2011, I went to the Moffitt Cancer Center in Tampa for the beginning of my stem cell therapy. I had to have a double lumen central IV catheter inserted for eventual use in harvesting and transfusing back my own stem cells. The catheter hung out of my left upper chest and was a real pain to take care of—it would be a companion for a long time.

The importance of the catheter can't be overstated, and to keep it fully functional it had to be irrigated regularly by personnel in Moffitt's BMT (Blood and Marrow Transplant) Unit. My stem cell transplant date was set for December 16, 2011. So, from October until then Lonni and I were at Moffitt every week to have catheter care in a private cubicle in the BMT Unit. I got to know all the nurses there very well (some of them had PhDs) during that time because it was a small unit and had virtually no turnover in personnel. Catheter care is a ritual performed using sterile technique and it took about half an hour.

On the last catheter irrigation session, before I went in for my transplant, Lonni and I met a nurse in the BMT Unit whom I'd *never* seen before. She was a light-complexioned black woman with just a hint of a Caribbean accent and not exquisitely well put together, like all the other nurses I knew—not scruffy, just not every hair in place. I was slightly uneasy as she went through the catheter care ritual and watched her like a hawk. She performed the procedure perfectly and was very friendly and professional in her demeanor.

When she finished, she came over and stood directly in front of me with an intense look on her face that was disquieting. The kind of look a person gives you when they seem to see something about/in you that you didn't even know about yourself. The best way to describe it is the kind of look somebody gives you when they know something that everybody knows except you, that commands your complete attention and is mildly disquieting.

She said, "Mr. Whitchurch, I know exactly what you are going to go through and I want to give you some advice. Eat when you don't want to, drink when you don't want to, and exercise when you don't want to, and you will be fine!"

I may have heard that advice before, but the way she said it burned it into my psyche and Lonni's too.

I left the BMT Unit, went into the hospital on December 14, 2011, had my transplant on December 16 and was discharged on December 31, weak as a kitten again.

In March 2012 I had to go back to the BMT Clinic at Moffitt for vaccinations to get my new immune system up to speed. I got my shots for DPT, measles, polio, tetanus, etc., etc. On my first visit back, I asked the secretary at the desk if the lady I'd last seen back in December for my last catheter irrigation was there. I wanted to thank her for that advice she gave me just before I went in. I didn't remember her name, but I described her: a light-complected black woman with a hint of a Caribbean accent and I pointed to the cubicle she'd treated me in.

The secretary looked puzzled and said she'd ask the head nurse who she was. The head nurse, whom I knew quite well, told me to describe her again which I did. She thought for a moment and said she wasn't sure whom I was referring to, so I started all over again. Midway through the first couple of words, she interrupted me and said, "Mr. Whitchurch, I know what you're saying but let me tell you, there's no one in this department who fits that description. As a matter of fact, there's never been anyone working in this department who fits that description, and I've been here for a long time." We were speechless.

Lonni and I left the department just staring at each other. It was powerful...

All the way home we talked about it in the car and I was emotionally wound tight. We couldn't come up with any explanation other than the obvious: She had just been there for me at that moment and had been sent by God to reassure, comfort, and guide me. An *angel*.

As I think back to those moments we spent together and remember the words she spoke, I dwell on her phraseology: "I know *exactly* what you are going to go through…. "Eat…drink…exercise…and *you will be fine!*" It made enough of an impression on me that I followed her advice to the letter. Those words stayed with me through my darkest moments, and I carry them in my heart now and consider them with the same reverence that Moses must have had for the words God spoke to him on Mount Sinai.

I only wish I could remember her name.

Below are two pictures (taken on an old flip phone camera, so they're kind of grainy) of me getting my stem cell transplant and how I looked when I finally came home after that ordeal. I had my University of Minnesota sweatpants on for the transplant occasion.

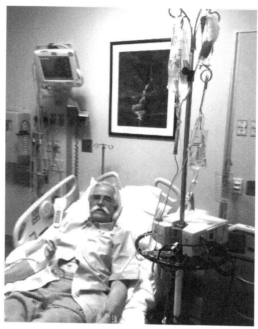

And here I am with Lonni on December 31, 2011.

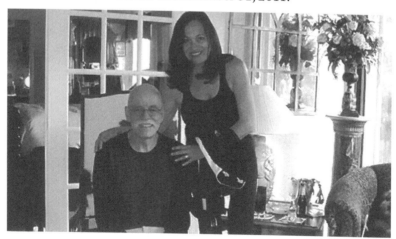

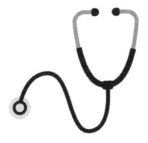

112. Room #4737

I was admitted to the BMT Unit at the Moffitt Cancer Center in Tampa, Florida, on December 14, 2011 for an autologous stem cell transplant. It was a fabulous room in a circular unit—mahogany cabinetry, couch, armchairs, and very spacious—like a luxury hotel room. I would be there for about three weeks or until my post-transplant blood work returned to acceptable levels. I had quite a few things with me to manage my life from that room and it took a while to get settled, get my computer set up, etc. I even liked the view and thought to myself, *What better place than this is there to go through everything?* I had a good sleep that night.

The next morning, my nurse came in and said that I'd have to change rooms. I really didn't want to since it would be a real pain to pack up again and move around the circle. She never gave me a good reason for the change; just said that she had received her orders from the head of the department and that I really didn't have a choice. There were plenty of unoccupied rooms on the ward and it made no sense to me but despite voicing my desire to stay put, I went along with the program.

I had high-dose chemo and the stem cell transplant and then drifted off into the vapors for the next couple weeks. Finally, my lab work was acceptable and a date for discharge was set.

I was to be discharged to a Marriot hotel, not far away from the hospital, which was specially equipped with a filtered air system for people like me with compromised immune systems and who needed quick access to the hospital in the event of a crisis. My lab work had to improve a little more to allow me to go home across the bay to Clearwater, Florida. A requirement for discharge was that I had to have a caregiver with me at all times (except when I was in Moffitt for a checkup) and an alternate caregiver available in the event my primary was unable to perform their function. My daughter Julie came down from Stillwater, Minnesota to be the primary so Lonni could take care of our house and our kitties and run the errands we needed her to do.

My daughter arrived at Moffitt the day of my discharge with Lonni and some friends, who had a large vehicle to fit all my stuff in. I met them at the entrance to my transplant unit and took everybody to my room. When my daughter saw the room number she gasped, clearly shocked and said, "*Oh, my god. Your room number is 4737!*" I said, "Yeah. So what?" "That's the house number of your mother's house in Minneapolis and the house she died in," she replied.

I'd been in that room almost three weeks and hadn't noticed.

I think it was more than coincidence that I had to change rooms for no apparent reason when I was admitted to Moffitt. I think it was a force from Heaven reaching down to let me know that my dear, sainted mother was there with me.

Everybody else thinks so too.

Below are pictures of my mother, Katherine Whitchurch, and her house in Minneapolis, MN.

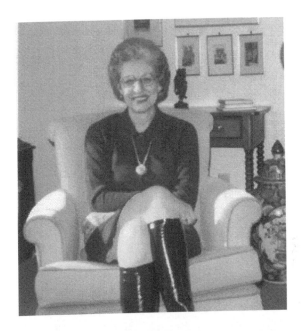

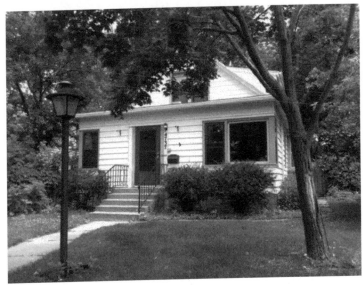

Glossary

AMBU: Artificial Mask Breathing Unit. A self-contained portable ventilating device **that** has a reservoir breathing bag that attaches to either a mask or endotracheal tube for portable ventilation of a patient

APGAR score: A measure of the physical condition of a newborn infant; **it** is obtained by adding points (2, 1, or 0) for heart rate, respiratory effort, muscle tone, response to stimulation, and skin coloration; **a** score of ten represents the best possible condition

Bronchoscopy: A procedure using a scope to examine the inside of the trachea, bronchi, and lungs

Craniotomy: Surgical opening into the skull

Cricoid pressure (Sellick maneuver): Associated with a rapid sequence induction of general anesthesia; **a** technique used during endotracheal intubation to reduce the risk of regurgitation; **it** involves the application of pressure to the cricoid cartilage in the neck, thus occluding the esophagus, which passes directly behind it

Cyanotic/Cyanosis: A bluish discoloration of the skin resulting from poor circulation or inadequate oxygenation of the blood

Debridement: A procedure for treating a wound in that involves cleaning and removing infected, non-viable (dead) tissue that may impede healing

DTs (delirium tremens): A psychotic condition typical of withdrawal in chronic alcoholics involving tremors, hallucinations, anxiety, and disorientation

Dyspnea: Difficult or labored breathing

Endotracheal tube: The tube placed into a patient's trachea for the purpose of ventilating them

Extubation: Removal of a tube from the trachea

Halothane: A volatile liquid anesthetic vaporized in a special calibrated vaporizer, mixed with oxygen and administered via an anesthesia machine to be inhaled by a patient, causing a state of surgical general anesthesia

Heimlich maneuver: A procedure employed to help a choking person who is conscious and unable to talk; it pushes air out of the person's lungs and makes him cough; the force of the cough may then move the object out of his airway; it involves wrapping your arms around the person's abdomen, from behind, placing your fist into the person's abdomen, and giving it a quick upward thrust

Innovar: The trade name of a potent narcotic and anti-psychotic/anti-emetic drug combination

Insufflation: The act of blowing anesthetic vapors into a patient's airway

Intubation with respect to airway management: Insertion of a tube into the trachea

IV: Intravenous

Laryngeal Mask Airway (LMA): A large endotracheal tube on the proximal end that connects to an elliptical mask on the distal end; designed to sit in the patient's hypopharynx and cover the supraglottic structures, thereby allowing relative isolation of the trachea

Laryngoscope: An instrument for close-up examination of the larynx used for inserting an endotracheal tube into the trachea

Laryngoscopy: An examination of your throat and larynx (voice box) with the use of a lighted instrument

Lateral dorsal recumbent position: The patient lying on their side, usually with their upper leg slightly flexed at the hip and knee and resting on a pillow.

Lavage: Washing out of a body cavity with normal saline or a medicated solution

Lithotomy position: A supine position of the body with the legs separated and elevated in stirrups

MAC anesthesia: Stands for Monitored Anesthesia Care; a type of procedure in which the patient has a local anesthetic supplemented by IV sedation and analgesia medications

MDA: Medical Doctor Anesthesiologist

Multiple Myeloma: A disease of the immune system in which the white blood cells in the bone marrow become cancerous and multiply

Oral airway: A device placed in an unconscious person's mouth to hold the tongue forward and keep the airway from becoming obstructed

Precordial: The portion of the body over the heart and lower chest

Tracheotomy: A surgical procedure to create an opening in the neck for direct access to the trachea

Yankauer suction handle (anesthesia): A tool used to suction oropharyngeal secretions in order to prevent airway obstruction and/or aspiration.

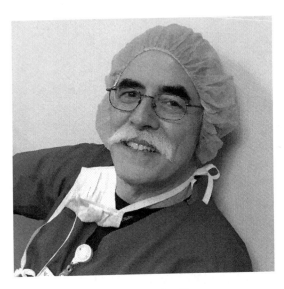

About the Author

I was born in South Bend, Indiana in September 1942. Shortly after that our family moved to Rockford, Illinois, where my father was an insurance executive and my mother was a housewife. Dad was transferred in 1946 and we moved to Minneapolis, where I grew up and was educated.

After high school I attended the University of Minnesota and pursued a course of study in mathematics, hoping someday to work for the government in the fledgling space program. While at the university, I worked part time as an orderly at one of the large Minneapolis city hospitals and loved it. I was especially fond of the times I was called to work in the operating room because I was right where the action was, especially at the head of the table with the Certified Registered Nurse Anesthetist (CRNA) and watching them make decisions about the patient's status during surgery and giving the drugs that kept them safe and asleep. The hospital had a nurse anesthesia program, and in talking to the CRNAs and students about their experiences, I was convinced that I needed to change my career plans and get into that field right away.

In June of 1966, after three years of mathematic studies, I left the university and entered the three year Registered Nursing diploma program at Abbott Hospital in Minneapolis. I ended up being the only male student in the class. I graduated in June 1969 and three months later passed my nursing boards to become a Registered Nurse. In November 1969 I was accepted into the nurse anesthesia program at the Minneapolis School of Anesthesia.

The anesthesia program at the Minneapolis School was eighteen months of morning clinicals, rotating to five large metropolitan hospitals, and three days a week of afternoon classes. After the first month we were allowed to do cases by ourselves with a CRNA there to help us start the case and available if we had any problems. We also took emergency calls with a CRNA for backup. It was probably one of the most well-rounded programs in existence then because the anesthesia departments at those hospitals all had different approaches and equipment to accomplish the same thing, which allowed me to see and employ many different techniques in administering anesthesia and served me well in the years that followed when I was alone doing emergency cases in the middle of the night.

After graduation I moved to Bemidji, Minnesota in 1971 with my wife and two young children. I went into practice with one other CRNA where we worked in a one hundred bed hospital doing all the anesthesia for scheduled and emergency call cases. Eventually we hired one full time and two part time CRNAs to split up the case load and calls. I stayed there for sixteen years, then moved to the Tampa Bay area of Florida in 1987 where I finished my career in a large, mixed group of anesthesiologists and CRNAs.

I thoroughly enjoyed my long, eventful career in the OR before I retired in 2018 at age 76. Now I am enjoying my retirement in Florida with my wife, Lonni.

Made in the USA
Columbia, SC
04 August 2021

42963052R00183